Writing for Capstone Projects and Publication in Occupational Therapy

This invaluable text explains how to compile and structure different forms of writing in occupational therapy, using easy-to-follow templates for capstone projects and publishable manuscripts.

Now aligned with the 7th edition of APA standards, the book can be used to help in the writing of needs assessments, case reports and case series, program evaluation, general research studies, intervention effectiveness studies, and instrument development and testing studies. This new edition also includes invaluable advice on writing a literature review, as well as harnessing artificial intelligence (AI) without invalidating a piece of writing. Embedded exercises assist readers to construct manuscripts step-by-step. The book also explains the publication process to guide readers to frame manuscripts in accordance with common publication expectations.

Illustrated with numerous examples throughout, and featuring essential guidance on both style and form, this is a wonderful resource whether you're a doctoral student writing as part of your capstone project, or an educator publishing for professional advancement.

Sharon A. Gutman held faculty positions in occupational therapy education programs for 30 years, including Columbia University (2006–2021) and Rutgers University (2021–2024) where she served as a full professor; she is currently retired. During her 30-year career, Dr. Gutman published 76 peer-reviewed journal articles, 14 textbooks, 26 textbook chapters, and 24 editorials. She was editor-in-chief of the *American Journal of Occupational Therapy* (AJOT) (2008–2014) and received the following professional awards: inducted into the American Occupational Therapy Association Roster of Fellows (2009); awarded the Cordelia Myers Best Paper in AJOT accolade (2021); and awarded the Eleanor Clarke Slagle Lectureship (2021).

Diane Powers Dirette is a professor in the Interdisciplinary Health Sciences PhD Program at Western Michigan University. She has published 19 peer-reviewed journal articles, 6 textbooks, 19 textbook chapters, and 37 editorials. Dr. Dirette is the co-founder and editor-in-chief of *The Open Journal of Occupational Therapy*. She has received the following professional awards: Teaching Excellence Award, CHHS, Western Michigan University (2003); Scholarship Excellence Award, CHHS, Western Michigan University (2014); American Occupational Therapy Association Roster of Fellows (2016); Hinojosa Distinguished Alumni Award, Department of OT, New York University (2020); and Michigan Occupational Therapy Association OT Award of Excellence, MiOTA (2023).

Writing for Capstone Projects and Publication in Occupational Therapy

Second Edition

Sharon A. Gutman and
Diane Powers Dirette

Routledge
Taylor & Francis Group
NEW YORK AND LONDON

Designed cover image: Routledge

Second edition published 2026
by Routledge
605 Third Avenue, New York, NY 10158

and by Routledge
4 Park Square, Milton Park, Abingdon, Oxon, OX14 4RN

Routledge is an imprint of the Taylor & Francis Group, an informa business

For Product Safety Concerns and Information please contact our EU representative GPSR@taylorandfrancis.com. Taylor & Francis Verlag GmbH, Kaufingerstraße 24, 80331 München, Germany.

First edition published by SLACK Incorporated 2017

ISBN: 978-1-041-22916-2 (hbk)
ISBN: 978-1-041-22869-1 (pbk)
ISBN: 978-1-003-73455-0 (ebk)

DOI: 10.4324/9781003734550

Typeset in Sabon
by Newgen Publishing UK

Contents

CHAPTER 1

Introduction

The Importance of Using Guidelines for Capstone Projects and Publishable Manuscripts

This book has two primary purposes: (a) to help entry-level and post-professional occupational therapy doctoral (OTD) students write their capstone projects in accordance with traditional reporting standard guidelines, and (b) to help new occupational therapy academic faculty to increase their chances of publication by preparing manuscripts for publication in accordance with traditional reporting standard guidelines.

Most OTD capstone projects at the entry- and post-professional levels fall into four categories: program evaluation, needs assessment, case report or case series, and general research studies (e.g., client satisfaction using survey design or interview).

Occupational therapy academic faculty commonly publish studies regarding intervention effectiveness, instrument development and testing, and exploratory studies examining clinical phenomena that have not previously been investigated.

All of these types of manuscripts should be written in accordance with specific reporting standards outlined by the health care community. This book is a compilation of the guidelines needed to report

- General research studies
- Intervention effectiveness studies
- Instrument development and testing studies
- Needs assessments
- Case reports and case series reports
- Program evaluations
- Discussion papers

In addition to the above writing guidelines, this book also provides chapters on

- Writing reviews of the literature
- Reporting statistical data in text and tables

DOI: 10.4324/9781003734550-1

Chapter 12 provides guidance about how to turn dissertations, capstone theses, and clinical data into publishable journal articles.

Chapters 13 through 17 provide guidance to help authors understand the publication process, including

- Preparing and submitting manuscripts for publication
- Writing manuscript cover letters
- The revision process
- Using AI in scholarly writing
- Ethical considerations in publication

Using the writing guidelines in this book will help entry- and post-professional-level OTD students to prepare their capstone project reports in a standard and efficient way. It will also assist occupational therapy faculty who are new to the publication process to prepare manuscripts that are congruent with publication expectations.

Readers should note that this book does not address the reporting of systematic reviews, as the reporting standards for these types of studies are detailed by the PRISMA standards, and readers are encouraged to use the materials generated by the Equator Network (2020).

Reference

Equator Network. (2020). *The PRISMA 2020 statement: An updated guideline for reporting systematic reviews*. www.equator-network.org/reporting-guidelines/prisma/

CHAPTER 2

Writing Resources

Mentors, Writing Partners, and Self-Discipline

Writing is an integral part of being an occupational therapy doctoral student or new academic faculty. Our success in these roles is measured by our ability to produce final written materials such as capstone project theses, published journal articles, books, research reports, and educational materials. While a command of English composition is a prerequisite, authors must also understand the differing style guidelines, formats, and objectives of the various written materials noted above. Each of these forms of written material requires different writing skill sets.

To obtain proficiency in writing skills, doctoral students and new academic faculty must engage in the process of reading examples from the literature and practicing writing by generating written drafts, obtaining feedback, and making revisions. To engage in this learning process, doctoral students and new faculty must continuously write and become emotionally neutral in response to feedback and critique. Feedback and critique should be used to strengthen drafts and should not be personalized. The process of redrafting, seeking feedback, and making revisions commonly requires multiple iterations.

Mentorship and Writing Support Groups

One of the most important resources when learning advanced writing skills is having one or more mentors who can provide feedback on multiple drafts until a paper is completed. Doctoral students traditionally gain assistance from an assigned faculty member who serves as a mentor in the development and completion of their capstone projects. New faculty can seek seasoned academicians as mentors who can provide guidance. Because academicians' workloads are often intense and they may not have time to mentor new faculty, it is sometimes beneficial for new faculty to offer paper coauthorship to secure mentorship. Doctoral students should acknowledge mentors in their capstone theses and offer coauthorship if the thesis becomes a published paper.

DOI: 10.4324/9781003734550-2

Doctoral students and new faculty can also form writing support groups in which they share their writing and receive constructive critique from their peers. Participating in writing support groups can feel less intimidating than requesting feedback from a seasoned academician; however, the critique offered may not be as valuable because the group members may have less experience in academic writing. Engaging in mentorship with a seasoned academic writer and participating in a writing support group are both highly recommended to help doctoral students and new faculty gain writing expertise.

Personal Commitment

While seasoned academic mentors and writing support groups are essential in the learning process, neither can enhance writing skills if doctoral students and new faculty do not make the commitment to write. To become a proficient academic writer, authors must engage in writing continuously. In other words, authors must devote a minimum of 3 hours per week to writing in one uninterrupted block of time. Attempting to write in smaller time periods will be unfruitful, because authors commonly need approximately 20 minutes to regain mental focus for a specific writing piece in order to begin writing where they last left off. Multitasking and writing are incompatible; doctoral students and new faculty must create a writing environment in which they are free from distractions such as cell phones, peers, colleagues, clients, family, and email. Creating a distraction-free writing environment and committing to a minimum 3-hour writing period per week require time management and self-discipline. A writing time period of 3 or more hours should be scheduled into the work/school week along with all other school- and work-related commitments. Honoring this scheduled time and adhering to this weekly schedule must become as sacrosanct as a covenant. To be a successful academic writer, doctoral students and new faculty must make a contract with themselves to devote the time needed to write.

The more authors adhere to a weekly writing schedule, the easier it becomes to sit down at a computer, free oneself from daily distractions, and regain the flow of writing. Each time that authors reschedule their weekly writing time period or make excuses to forgo a writing session, the more difficult it becomes to regain writing flow. Soon the thought of writing becomes a distasteful chore that is consistently avoided, and writing projects become abandoned or hastily completed to meet rapidly approaching due dates.

Decreasing Writing Anxiety

One way that doctoral students and new faculty can prevent writing anxiety and avoidance is to outline all writing projects at the beginning and create a map or set of instructions that can be followed at each writing session. At the end of each writing session, authors should make notes to themselves about how to restart writing and identify the next writing steps. The day or evening prior to their next scheduled writing session, authors should read their previous notes to direct their mental focus back to the writing project. Sleeping with those notes and directions in mind and then embarking upon writing the next day will help authors ease back into their writing.

Sometimes having a writing partner effectively helps authors commit to a weekly writing schedule and set and meet deadlines. A writing partner can be a student or colleague who is similarly involved in their own writing projects. Writing partners can schedule appointments together to write at the library (or another quiet environment), and they can act as coaches to make sure that each author is setting and adhering to deadlines.

Doctoral students and new faculty must also depersonalize feedback and recognize that it pertains to a set of sentences on a page rather than to themselves. It is also beneficial to recognize that articles are published in a polished form after multiple drafts, revisions, and professional editing. Authors must remember that first drafts, even those written by seasoned writers, often read very differently from final papers ready for publication. The more comfortable we become sharing our preliminary drafts with others, the more feedback we will receive that can ultimately help us reach publication readiness. The more we write, the less anxiety writing will cause us.

Checklist for Gathering and Using Writing Resources

- ☐ Read the professional literature to gain an understanding of the writing styles and formats that characterize the types of materials you wish to write.
- ☐ Understand that writing a paper involves the development of multiple drafts, seeking feedback for each draft, and making several sets of revisions. This is a lengthy process, and one writing project can require weeks or months for completion.
- ☐ Seek a mentor who is a seasoned academic writer with a strong publication history and who can provide feedback on drafts of your written material. Doctoral students should acknowledge mentors in their capstone theses and offer coauthorship if the thesis becomes a published paper. New faculty can offer coauthorship on published papers to seasoned academic writers who serve as mentors.
- ☐ Participate in a writing support group with academic colleagues who are similarly seeking to develop writing skills in a supportive environment.
- ☐ Commit to a weekly writing schedule of 3-hour or greater blocks. Schedule this writing period into your work/school week and adhere to it.
- ☐ Avoid multitasking during your 3-hour weekly writing session. Write in a nondistracting environment free of cell phones, email, and interruptions.
- ☐ Outline all writing projects before beginning to write. At the end of each writing session, make notes or a set of directions that will help you restart writing at your next scheduled session.
- ☐ The day or night before each scheduled writing session, review your notes so that your mind begins to regain focus on the project while you sleep. Begin writing again the next day.
- ☐ If you have difficulty with self-discipline and avoid writing, seek a writing partner who is similarly either a new academician with the objective of a writing career or a doctoral student who is completing their capstone thesis. Schedule writing sessions together and help each other set and adhere to writing deadlines.
- ☐ Depersonalize feedback and become comfortable receiving critique on written drafts. Recognize that preliminary drafts read very differently from final, publication-ready papers that have gone through multiple drafts, revisions, and professional editing.

CHAPTER 3

Writing Reviews of the Literature

A literature review is a critical analysis of the research on a specific topic that provides the reader with a synthesis or summary of the existing body of knowledge. A literature review may be conducted to elucidate the gaps in existing research, to understand how a concept is defined and used in a profession, to determine the scope and adequacy of available studies on a topic, or to synthesize evidence relevant to a particular practice. This chapter defines and discusses four types of literature reviews: narrative reviews, concept analyses, scoping reviews, and systematic reviews.

Narrative Reviews

Narrative reviews are an examination of the existing research literature related to a topic. Although some narrative reviews are free-standing manuscripts, this guide is for the literature review section of a research manuscript. In research manuscripts, following the background and definitions of a problem, researchers write a narrative that describes the recent, relevant research related to the topic of study. In other words, this section tells the reader what research has already been done on the topic. The review of the literature should elucidate the knowledge gap that the current study will address and should end with the research questions or hypotheses.

The various ways a narrative review can be organized include historical, thematic, dichotomous, or methodological, depending on the existing research being reviewed. A historical literature review presents the development of research chronologically, discussing the research over time. A thematic literature review groups research according to key topics or issues. A dichotomous review presents two different viewpoints on a topic. A methodological review is organized according to the research designs that were used in the studies.

The following highlights the main parts of a narrative review, including the introduction, body, and conclusion. Authors should introduce the research literature; organize, critique, and synthesize the information; and draw logical conclusions that lead to the

DOI: 10.4324/9781003734550-3

research questions or hypotheses of the current study. By the end of the literature review, the need to answer the research questions should be apparent.

Writing Exercises: Narrative Reviews

- Use key search words to gather all the recent, relevant research related to your topic.
- Identify the type of organization you will use based on the research that is available on this topic (e.g., historical, thematic).
- Write an outline of your narrative review based on your decided organization.
- List the strengths of the research you reviewed.
- List the limitations (stated and unstated) of the research you reviewed.
- Summarize the implications for further research stated by the authors of the research.
- Use the limitations and implications for further research to write a statement about how your research will address one or more of the research gaps and contribute to the body of knowledge.

Checklist for Writing Narrative Reviews

Introduction

☐ Explain the overall topic, purpose, and organization of the literature review.

Body

☐ Present and critique the research for content or methodological strengths and limitations.
☐ Synthesize information from multiple sources to identify patterns, trends, and relationships, rather than just summarizing each source individually.
☐ Use subheadings to break down the body into logical sections based on the chosen organization.

Conclusion

☐ Summarize the main points of the literature review, highlighting trends, conflicts, and gaps.
☐ Explain how the current study will address these gaps and contribute to the body of knowledge.
☐ State the research questions or hypotheses of the current study.

Concept Analyses

Concepts are clusters of attributes related to a phenomenon that are the core building blocks of theories. Concept analysis is a form of inquiry used to identify, clarify, refine, and advance the understanding of a phenomenon to develop and expand the knowledge base of a profession (Rodgers & Knafl, 2000). Concept analysis is used to synthesize existing knowledge about a concept, enhance communication about phenomena, and provide for categorization of phenomena, such as the development of taxonomies.

General types of concept analysis may include examinations of various points of view, the historical development of a concept, or the philosophy regarding a concept. An examination of the history of a concept may help elucidate how scientific advancements have changed the understanding of the phenomenon, the underlying theory, or the terminology that is used. For example, as instruments have been developed that help neuroscientists explain brain function, our understanding of phenomena such as the underlying attributes of mental conditions has advanced, and concepts related to these phenomena can be better described and delineated using concept analyses.

Concept analyses address internal or external issues. An internal issue is a problem with clarity regarding the aspects, attributes, or levels that constitute the concept. Different authors may provide varied views on what aspects, attributes, or levels constitute a concept. For example, the levels of what constitutes self-awareness may be based on differing theoretical perspectives. Some authors may state that self-awareness progresses from intellectual to anticipatory levels of understanding based on clinical observations, while others may state that self-awareness progresses from concrete to abstract based on the neurological components that correlate with self-awareness. Sansonetti et al. (2025) provide an excellent example of a concept analysis of online awareness.

An external issue is a problem with the use of varied labels and definitions for the same concept. External concept analyses help to resolve conceptual problems, such as nebulous or vague terminology or overlapping attributes of a concept. For example, there are varied perspectives on the concepts that are labeled as post-traumatic stress disorder and complex trauma. Some authors use those labels as separate concepts, while others use them as the same concept. A concept analysis would clarify these concepts to improve the understanding of the attributes that are overlapping or different to determine if these are the same or different concepts. Some concept analyses may be both internal and external, developing an understanding of the attributes of a concept and also clarifying what makes that concept different from other conceptualizations of a phenomenon. The steps for conducting concept analyses are based in part on Rodgers (2000).

Steps for Conducting Concept Analyses

1. Identify the concept of interest and potential alternative labels for that concept.
2. Formulate a research question based on a preliminary search of the literature.
3. Determine if the purpose of the study is an examination of internal, external, or both.
4. Develop a protocol and define inclusion, exclusion, and literature search criteria.
5. Conduct a thorough and systematic search of relevant literature using the criteria.
6. Develop a data charting form or grid for systematic data collection of the attributes of the concepts or the varied labels.
7. Collect the data from the full-text articles with at least two researchers reaching an agreement.
8. Analyze the data using inductive and qualitative thematic analyses.
9. Identify an exemplar of the concept or distinguishing features of concepts.

10. Discuss the implications, hypotheses, and any need for further development of the concept.

Concept analysis should be a continual process and conducted periodically as advanced theoretical knowledge is developed. For example, Cowles and Rodgers (2000) provide a concept analysis of grief. In this example, the authors explore both the internal attributes that constitute grief and how grief compares to the external labels of bereavement and mourning. Future concept analyses could examine how advances in neurological and physiological knowledge about the underlying bodily changes that occur in grief further explain the internal attributes that constitute the concept of grief.

Writing Exercises: Concept Analyses

- List all possible labels for the concept being analyzed.
- Conduct a preliminary search for the definitions of these concepts.
- List the preliminary findings, including the labels and the attributes that you found.
- If the attributes of the concept are not well defined, conduct an internal concept analysis.
- If the concepts seem to be the same but different labels are used, or if there is overlap in attributes, conduct an external concept analysis.

Checklist for Writing Concept Analyses

Title

☐ Include the concept or concepts being analyzed.
☐ Identify the study as a concept analysis in the title.

Introduction

☐ Describe the historical or philosophical issues related to this concept.
☐ State the problem (internal, external, or both).
☐ Discuss the theoretical differences underlying the problem.

Method

☐ State the purpose, sampling design, and data collection methods.
☐ Detail the search terms and resources that were used to acquire literature.
☐ Indicate the quantitative and qualitative descriptive analyses that will be used.

Results

☐ Present the literature from a historical, theoretical, or philosophical perspective as appropriate to the problem.

- ☐ Analyze and synthesize the literature. Concept analyses may include statistics on the prevalence of use, qualitative meta-ethnography (thematic, inductive integration of qualitative results), concept mapping, or a combination of these analyses.

Discussion

- ☐ Interpret the findings. Discuss the attributes that make up the concept (internal) or distinguish one concept from another (external).
- ☐ Discuss implications for health care professionals, limitations of the analysis, and implications for further research.

Scoping Reviews

A scoping review is the selection, collection, and synthesis of the literature to identify, map, and summarize the available evidence related to assessment, intervention, or policy. The scoping review may examine the breadth, depth, and methods of the research to identify gaps in knowledge related to a particular topic and to provide implications for further research (Levac et al., 2010; Munn et al., 2018). In general, the purposes of scoping reviews are exploratory and descriptive (Peters et al., 2020).

The specific purpose of a scoping review may include one or more of the following.

- ☐ Summarize the amount and extent of research on a specific topic.
- ☐ Map the literature to identify the gaps in existing knowledge.
- ☐ Collect and synthesize the available assessments for a specific problem.
- ☐ Analyze the psychometrics that support assessments for a specific population or context.
- ☐ Synthesize and summarize the amount of available evidence to inform practice or policymaking.
- ☐ Identify and map the policies that impact practice in a particular area.
- ☐ Investigate the methods used to examine the effectiveness of an intervention or policy.
- ☐ Analyze the quality of the available evidence to support intervention or policy.
- ☐ Provide implications for further research.
- ☐ Determine the need for and feasibility of a systematic review.

Scoping reviews are guided by specific research aims or questions. The research question or aim should include the population, concept, and context (PCC) to help guide the inclusion criteria and literature search (Peters et al., 2020). For example, a research question to collect and synthesize available assessments might be "What instruments are available to assess independence, safety, and function for individuals residing in assisted living facilities?" In an example from the occupational therapy literature, Berg et al. (2022) conducted a scoping review guided by the research question "What is the evidence in relation to the use of Masgutova Neurosensorimotor Reflex Integration (MNRI®) as a therapeutic intervention?" In this study, the authors found that the research regarding MNRI® lacked rigor, was conducted only by individuals affiliated with the creator of the treatment, and did not use assessments with known psychometric properties, leading to their conclusion that the efficacy of this treatment cannot be established and that independent research is needed. In another scoping review, Lucus Molitor et al. (2023) aimed to map the available literature on the types of occupation-based interventions provided to women with breast cancer. Because of a lack of available research, the authors concluded that there is a need for more research regarding occupation-based occupational therapy interventions for women with breast cancer.

Guidelines for Scoping Reviews

Scoping reviews have become a more common methodological choice for researchers (Peters et al., 2020). To improve the methodological rigor of scoping reviews, several guidelines have been developed for conducting the research and reporting findings. In their seminal work, Arksey and O'Malley (2005) presented a framework for conducting scoping reviews, and several authors have further developed and refined those guidelines (Colquhoun et al., 2014; Levac et al., 2010; Peters et al., 2020). The steps for conducting scoping reviews outlined in this chapter are a compilation of information from these sources.

In addition to these guidelines for conducting scoping reviews, the PRISMA extension for scoping reviews (PRISMA-ScR) (Tricco et al., 2018) provides guidelines for reporting the results of scoping reviews. The PRISMA-ScR checklist contains 20 essential reporting items and 2 optional items to include when reporting a scoping review. The 20 essential items guide the title, abstract, introduction, methods, results, discussion, and funding reporting. The two optional items relate to the critical appraisal of individual sources of evidence, as this is not completed in all scoping reviews. For the results section, it is recommended that researchers use the PRISMA flow diagram (see Figure 3.1) to elucidate the screening process.

Steps for Conducting Scoping Reviews

1. Formulate a research question using a framework such as PCC.
2. Determine the purpose of the study.
3. Develop a protocol and define inclusion, exclusion, and search criteria.
4. Conduct a thorough and systematic search of relevant literature using the criteria.
5. Screen and select studies using an iterative process of searching, refining, and reviewing articles. At least two researchers should determine the selection of articles to be included. Use a third researcher to resolve disagreements.
6. Develop a data charting form or grid for systematic data collection of the needed variables or information from the selected articles that will be used to answer the research question.
7. Collect the data from the full-text articles with at least two researchers reaching an agreement.
8. Analyze the data using descriptive numerical summary analyses and qualitative thematic analyses.
9. Critically appraise the quality of the studies using standardized tools or checklists to ensure a consistent and objective assessment. (Optional)
10. Report on the results related to the research question.

11. Discuss and interpret the findings related to the purpose of the study.
12. Identify the limitations of the study.
13. Determine the implications for practice, policy, and/or further research.
14. Consider using consultation from agencies, consumers, stakeholders, and therapists to further understand the phenomenon. Report any findings from consultations.

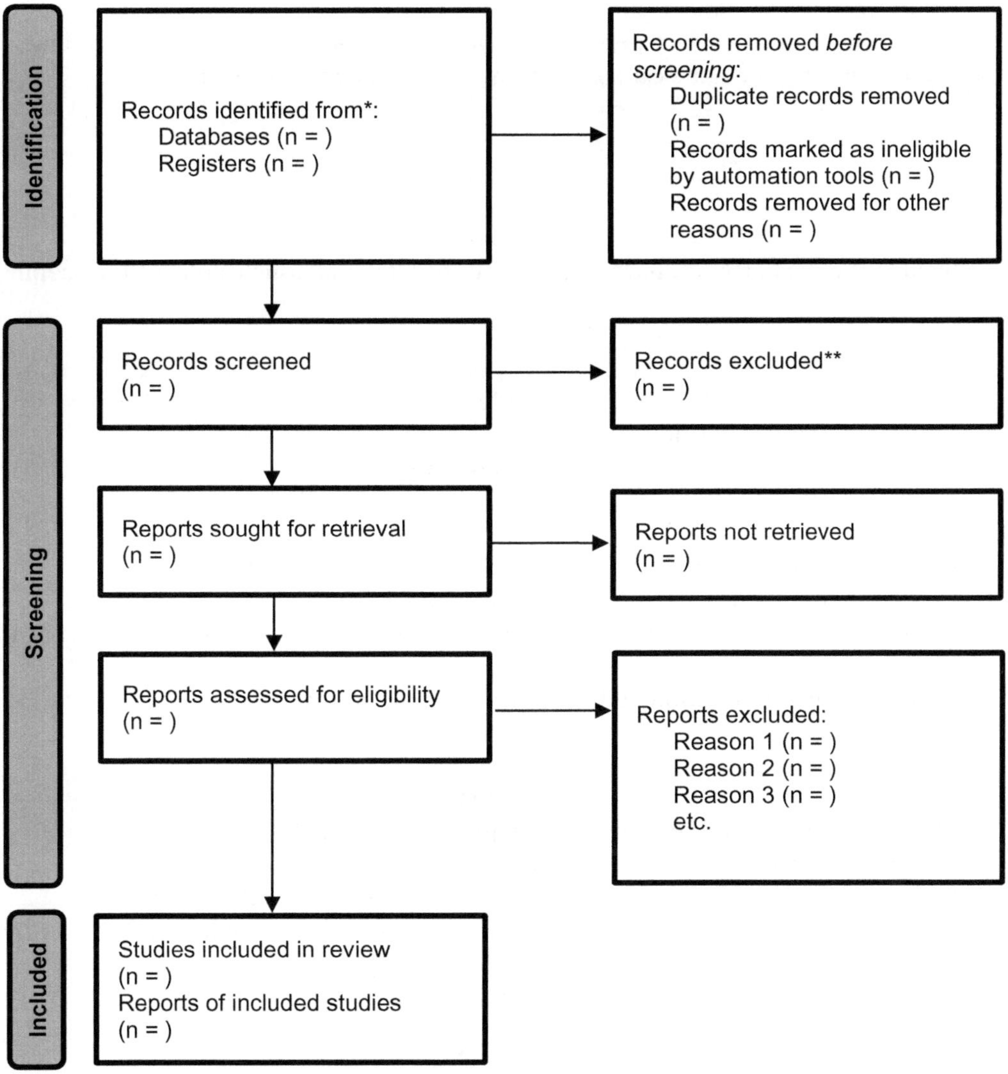

Figure 3.1 PRISMA Flow Diagram

*Consider, if feasible to do so, reporting the number of records identified from each database or register searched (rather than the total number across all databases/registers).

**If automation tools were used, indicate how many records were excluded by a human and how many were excluded by automation tools.

Writing Exercises: Scoping Reviews

- Identify the population, concepts, and context (PCC).
- Write a title using the PCC and the words "scoping review."
- Read the title to a person unfamiliar with your study to assess the ability of your title to convey the content of your manuscript.
- Write the abstract using one to two sentences to summarize your background, purpose, method, results, and conclusion.
- Read the abstract to two people, one who is familiar with your study and one who is not, to assess the clarity and completeness of your abstract.

Checklist for Writing Scoping Reviews

Abstract

☐ Include the background, purpose, method, results, and conclusions of the scoping review.

Title

☐ Use PCC to write the title.
☐ Identify the study as a scoping review in the title.

Introduction

☐ Present the background of the problem that is being addressed.
☐ Introduce and define each of the variables in the scoping review.
☐ Discuss what is already known about the problem in relation to the variables and context.
☐ State the research question and the purpose of the study.

Method

☐ Identify the design of the study and the justification for the design.
☐ State the inclusion, exclusion, and search criteria.
☐ Describe the protocol and procedures that were used to search the literature.
☐ Provide the rationale and criteria for critical appraisal, if completed as part of the study.
☐ Indicate the data analysis plan that was developed.

Results

☐ Present the screening process that was completed, preferably using the PRISMA Flow Diagram.
☐ Describe the characteristics of the data that were collected and charted related to the research question/s (may include a table).

- ☐ If completed, present the critical appraisal of the studies that were included.
- ☐ Synthesize the results to conclude the section.

Discussion

- ☐ Interpret the results to answer the research questions.
- ☐ Compare the results to the background information in the study and explain any differences using the available literature.
- ☐ Identify any limitations of the scoping review.
- ☐ Provide a conclusion that summarizes the findings and discusses implications for practice, policy, and further research.

Systematic Reviews

A systematic review is an analysis and synthesis of the available literature that answers research questions about the quality of the evidence regarding assessment, intervention, or policy. Systematic reviews help guide evidence-based practice by identifying the quality, quantity, and level of evidence available for use in a profession. Systematic reviews may identify and investigate conflicting results to elucidate and clarify the available evidence. And finally, systematic reviews may provide and inform areas for future research (Munn et al., 2018). Meta-analyses are often conducted to integrate the statistical findings of the research articles. Prior to conducting a systematic review, researchers may consider conducting a scoping review to determine the availability of experimental research studies and the feasibility of completing meta-analyses of the findings.

Ultimately, systematic reviews answer specific research aims or questions that help guide practice. Systematic reviews form the basis of evidence-based practice and help determine the need for further research. For example, Pacheco et al. (2025) conducted a systematic review of the literature to critically evaluate the existing evidence from randomized controlled trials that target physical activity, sedentary behaviors, and sleep to understand their effects on cognitive outcomes in early childhood. By synthesizing findings from high-quality studies, these researchers were able to determine that physical activity interventions, particularly those involving cognitively engaging activities, significantly improved cognitive domains such as executive function, inhibition, and attention while also determining the need for further research on integrated interventions that address physical activity, sedentary behaviors, and sleep.

Guidelines for Systematic Reviews

Two well-established resources help guide systematic reviews, including the Cochrane Handbook for Systematic Reviews of Interventions (Higgins et al., 2019) and the Preferred Reporting Items for Systematic Reviews and Meta-Analysis (PRISMA) 2020 statement for reporting systematic reviews and meta-analyses (www.prisma-statement.org/prisma-2020). The Cochrane Handbook for Systematic Reviews of Interventions provides guidelines for specific, high-quality systematic reviews. Not all systematic reviews will be Cochrane reviews. The guidelines, however, are useful as a basis for finding, appraising, and synthesizing evidence to answer specific research questions.

PRISMA guides the researcher on reporting the findings from the systematic reviews and meta-analyses to improve transparency and quality. PRISMA includes a 27-item checklist for the main report, a 12-item checklist for the abstract, and a flow diagram to visually track the number of studies included and excluded and the reasons for exclusion. The 27-item list details the essential reporting elements that should be included in each section of the manuscript, including the title, abstract, introduction, methods, results, and discussion sections. The flow diagram is a visual template that illustrates the flow of information through the review process, from initial identification of records to the final included studies. Different templates are available for new vs. updated reviews (see Figure 3.1).

Steps for Conducting Systematic Reviews

1. Formulate a research question using a framework such as PCC.
2. Identify the purpose of the study.
3. Develop a protocol and define the criteria.
4. Conduct a thorough and systematic search of relevant literature across multiple databases to find all eligible studies.
5. Screen and select studies based on the inclusion and exclusion criteria.
6. Critically appraise the quality of the studies using standardized tools or checklists to ensure a consistent and objective assessment.
7. Systematically extract relevant data from each included study and synthesize the findings from all included studies, which may involve a narrative summary or a meta-analysis to combine the results statistically.
8. Summarize the evidence and interpret the findings.

Writing Exercises: Systematic Reviews

- List the databases you will use to search for articles.
- Identify your key search terms.
- Identify the context of the search (e.g., geographical boundaries, language of publication).
- Complete the PRISMA diagram and have a researcher review it to ensure that the reasons for exclusion are clear.
- Write your meta-analysis process in a clear step-by-step description. Consult with a statistician to review your meta-analyses to assess the accuracy of your analyses and the clarity of your description.
- Write a conclusion section and compare it to your introduction paragraph and research question to ensure that it matches the initial purpose and answers the research question clearly and concisely.

Checklist for Writing Systematic Reviews

Abstract

- ☐ Include the background, purpose, method, results, and conclusions of the systematic review.

Title

- ☐ Use PCC to write the title.
- ☐ Identify the study as a systematic review in the title.

Introduction

- ☐ Discuss the background of the problem being addressed (assessment, intervention, or policy).
- ☐ Introduce and define each of the variables in the systematic review.
- ☐ Review the relevant literature regarding the problem being addressed.
- ☐ Clearly state a question that the systematic review will answer.

Method

- ☐ Identify the design.
- ☐ Define the inclusion/exclusion criteria.
- ☐ Explain the search strategies and screening of articles.
- ☐ Detail the data analysis plan.

Results

- ☐ Identify the articles that were used in the study using the PRISMA diagram.
- ☐ Report the results using narrative summary and meta-analyses.

Discussion

- ☐ Interpret the findings and the implications for practice.
- ☐ Discuss the limitations and implications for further research.

References

Arksey, H., & O'Malley, L. (2005). Scoping studies: Towards a methodological framework. *International Journal of Social Research Methodology, 8*(1), 19–32. https://doi.org/10.1080/1364557032000119616

Berg, L. A., Brown, D., Kroll, K., Pfaff, C., & Cleveland, L. (2022). The Masgutova Neurosensorimotor Reflex Integration (MNRI®): A scoping review. *Open Journal of Occupational Therapy, 10*(4), 1–16.

Colquhoun, H. L., Levac, D., O'Brien, K. K., Straus, S., Tricco, A. C., Perrier, L., Kastner, M., & Moher, D. (2014). Scoping reviews: Time for clarity in definition, methods, and reporting. *Journal of Clinical Epidemiology, 67*(12), 1291–1294. https://doi.org/10.1016/j.jclinepi.2014.03.013

Cowles, K. V., & Rodgers, B. L. (2000). The concept of grief. In Rodgers, B., & Knafl, K. (Eds.), *Concept development in nursing: Foundations, techniques, and applications* (2nd ed.). Sauders.

Higgins, J. P. T., Thomas, J., Chandler, J., Cumpston, M., Li, T., Page, M. J., & Welch, V. A. (2019). *Cochrane handbook for systematic reviews of interventions* (2nd ed.). Wiley.

Levac, D., Colquhoun, H., & O'Brien, K. K. (2010). Scoping studies: Advancing the methodology. *Implementation Science: IS*, *5*(1), 69–69. https://doi.org/10.1186/1748-5908-5-69

Lucas Molitor, W., Clark, E., & Moser, B. (2023). A scoping review of occupation-based Interventions for women with breast cancer. *Open Journal of Occupational Therapy, 11*(1), 1–9. https://doi.org/10.15453/2168-6408.2046

Munn, Z., Peters, M., Stern, C., McArthur, A., & Aromataris, E. (2018). Systematic review or scoping review? Guidance for authors when choosing between a systematic or scoping review approach. *BMC Medical Research Methodology, 18*(143), 1–7. https://doi.org/10.1186/s12874-018-0611-x

Pacheco, C., Culkin, V., Putkaradze, A., & Zang, N. (2025). Effects of movement behaviors on preschoolers' cognition: A systematic review of randomized controlled trials. *International Journal of Behavioral Nutrition and Physical Activity, 22*(12). https://doi.org/10.1186/s12966-025-01705-y

Peters, M. D. J., Marnie, C., Tricco, A. C., Pollock, D., Munn, Z., Alexander, L., McInerney, P., Godfrey, C. M., & Khalil, H. (2020). Updated methodological guidance for the conduct of scoping reviews. *JBI Evidence Synthesis, 18*(10), 2119–2126. https://doi.org/10.11124/JBIES-20-00167

Rodgers, B. (2000). Concept analysis: An evolutionary view. In Rodgers, B., & Knafl, K. (Ed.), *Concept development in nursing: Foundations, techniques, and applications* (2nd ed., pp. 77–102). Saunders.

Rodgers, B. L., & Knafl, K. A. (2000). Introduction to concept development in nursing. In Rodgers, B., & Knafl, K. (Ed.), *Concept development in nursing: Foundations, techniques, and applications* (2nd ed.). Sauders.

Sansonetti, D., Fleming, J., Patterson, F., Lannin, N. A., & Toglia, J. (2025). Online awareness: A concept analysis and review of assessment approaches for adults with neurological conditions. *Disability and Rehabilitation*, *47*(2), 324–339. https://doi.org/10.1080/09638288.2024.2338876

Tricco, A. C., Lillie, E., Zarin, W., O'Brien, K. K., Colquhoun, H., Levac, D., ... & Straus, S. E. (2018). PRISMA extension for scoping reviews (PRISMA-ScR): Checklist and explanation. *Annals of Internal Medicine*, *169*(7), 467–473. https://doi.org/10.7326/M18-0850

CHAPTER 4

Manuscript Structure and Content for General Research Studies

This section reviews in depth the basic content and structure of a research paper. The term *general research studies* refers to basic research and nonexperimental designs such as descriptive, qualitative, correlational, survey, longitudinal, and cross-sectional. A primary concern for publishers is the cost of publication space. Even online publication has costs associated with copyediting and journal website maintenance. General manuscript length requirements are usually 5,000 words, including references; however, it is critical to check the page and word count lengths in the author guidelines of the specific journal to which you intend to submit and adhere to those requirements. Not adhering to journal page length and word count will often result in returned manuscripts.

Research manuscripts for health care journals and capstone projects should be written concisely and use the least amount of words to convey clear, in-depth meaning. There is a specific formula for writing research manuscripts that most editors and reviewers seek. Writing your research manuscript in accordance with this formatting structure will ensure that you have addressed the critical elements needed to clearly and transparently describe your study methodology and report results. If a journal's author guidelines diverge from the following formatting structure, authors should use the structure recommended by the journal. If no structure is provided in the journal's author guidelines, use the following structure (whose heading levels are based on the *Publication Manual of the American Psychological Association*, 7th edition [American Psychological Association, 2020]). The following headings are provided for a masked manuscript, or one in which the authors' identifying information and affiliated institutions are removed.

DOI: 10.4324/9781003734550-4

Manuscript Headings and Formatting for General Research Studies

Title

Begin the manuscript with a title on a separate title page. The title should be centered, bolded, and typed in uppercase and lowercase letters.

Abstract

The Abstract should be placed on the page directly following the title page. The word *Abstract* should be capitalized, centered, and bolded. If keywords are required, they are inserted directly after the abstract and indented. The term *keywords* is italicized, capitalized, and indented:

Keywords: stroke, community participation, activities of daily living

Introduction

The Introduction begins on the page directly following the Abstract. The heading *Introduction* is not typed in the manuscript because the beginning of the manuscript text alerts the reader that the Introduction has begun.

Literature Review

Literature reviews can be (a) embedded within the Introduction without a separate subheading; (b) embedded in the Introduction with a separate subheading that is bolded, capitalized, and flush left; or (c) inserted following the Introduction as a separate section with a heading that is bolded, capitalized, and centered.

Method

The Method section is positioned directly after the Introduction. The heading *Method* is capitalized, centered, and bolded.

Research Design

Research Design is the first subheading in the Method section. It is bolded, capitalized, and flush left.

Participants

Participants is the second subheading in the Method section. It is bolded, capitalized, and flush left.

Instruments

Instruments is commonly the third subheading in the Method section. It is bolded, capitalized, and flush left.

Procedures

Procedures is commonly the fourth subheading in the Method section. It is bolded, capitalized, and flush left.

Data Collection

Data Collection is the subheading that directly follows the Procedures section. It is bolded, capitalized, and flush left.

Data Analysis

Data Analysis is the subheading that directly follows the Data Collection section. It is bolded, capitalized, and flush left.

Results

The Results section directly follows the Data Analysis section and begins a new section of the manuscript. The heading *Results* is bolded, centered, and capitalized.

Discussion

The Discussion section directly follows the Results and begins a new section of the manuscript. The heading *Discussion* is bolded, centered, and capitalized.

Limitations

The Limitations subsection is part of the Discussion section but should be highlighted for the reader by a separate subheading. The subheading *Limitations* is bolded, capitalized, and flush left.

Future Research

The Future Research subsection directly follows the Limitations subsection. This section is also part of the Discussion and should be highlighted for the reader by a separate subheading. The subheading *Future Research* is bolded, capitalized, and flush left.

Implications for Practice

Implications for Practice is a subsection of the Discussion section and follows the Future Research section. The subheading *Implications for Practice* is bolded, capitalized, and flush left.

Conclusion

The Conclusion is the final subsection of the Discussion and follows Implications for Practice. The heading is bolded, capitalized, and flush left.

References

References begin on a separate page following the Conclusion. The heading is centered, capitalized, and bolded.

Tables

Tables should be provided after the end of the references and should begin on a separate page. Each table should be presented on its own page. Tables are named and presented in accordance with the order in which they are mentioned in the text. The title of the Table is inserted beneath the Table heading:

Table 1 [bolded, capitalized, and flush left]
Participant Demographics [italicized, capitalized, and flush left]

Figures

Figures should be provided after the end of the tables and begin on a separate page. Each figure should be presented on its own page. Figures are named and presented in accordance with the order in which they are mentioned in the text. The title of the Figure is inserted beneath the Figure heading:

Figure 1 [bolded, capitalized, and flush left]
Examples of Participant Quotes [italicized, capitalized, and flush left]

Manuscript Heading Content for General Research Studies

There should be no repetition of content in the manuscript. The following sections and subsections should not contain overlap, which they will not if written as suggested.

Title

Titles help indexers categorize articles so that they can be easily accessed. If critical information is missing from titles, articles may never be accessed by their intended audience. The title of general research manuscripts should concisely describe the topic and identify the main variables examined. Titles should contain the following elements:

- The population addressed
- The independent variable (or topical issue addressed)
- The dependent variable (or topical issue addressed)
- The research design

Examples of good research manuscript titles include the following:

- Relationship Between Pencil Grasp and Handwriting Precision in 1st Graders With ADHD
- Factors That Facilitate and Impede Transition to Housing in the Chronically Homeless: A Phenomenological Study
- A Survey of Program Director Perceptions About Transitioning to OTD Entry-Level Programs

Abbreviations in titles should be avoided unless commonly used and understood in the health care community.

Writing Exercises: Titles

- Practice writing a title for your manuscript or capstone project using the above guidelines.
- For a quantitative study, identify the population, independent and dependent variables, and research design. Ensure that all of these appear in the title.
- For a qualitative study, identify the population, qualitative variable addressed, and research design. Ensure that all of these appear in the title.
- Ask a peer to read your title and describe what they think your paper is about. If they are correct, you have likely written an adequate title. If they are not correct, you may need to revise your title using the above directions.

Abstract

Unless otherwise specified by a journal's author guidelines, general research manuscripts and capstone projects should summarize the paper content using the abstract subheadings (a) objectives, (b) method, (c) results, and (d) conclusions. Using these subheadings will ensure that you provide the reader with critical information needed to understand paper content and select papers from database searches. Although most abstracts are between 150 and 200 words, authors should check and adhere to the word count specifications outlined in a journal's author guidelines.

- Objectives: In one to two sentences, authors should describe the purpose of the study.
- Method: In one to two sentences, authors should provide information about participants (e.g., population, sample size, recruitment strategies), research design, and data collection procedures.
- Results: In one to two sentences, authors should report the primary findings along with statistical test results and exact p values. Report confidence intervals alongside p values to provide a measure of the effect size and its precision.
- Conclusions: In one to two sentences, authors should describe the implications of their study for the clinical population and profession.

Writing Exercises: Abstracts [approximately 150–200 words]

- See the example papers at the end of this chapter to gain a clearer understanding of how to write abstracts.
- The abstract is the last section that should be written after all other manuscript sections are completed.

- Practice writing an abstract for your manuscript or capstone project using the following guidelines.
- Objectives: Go to the purpose statement of your manuscript and identify the purpose of the paper. Modify this sentences(s) so that it is not taken verbatim from the manuscript text.
- Method: Go to your Methods section of your manuscript and identify information regarding the following: participants (e.g., population, sample size, recruitment), research design, and data collection procedures. Revise these sentences so that they are not written verbatim and can be shortened and combined into one to two sentences.
- Results: Select the primary findings from your Results section. You will likely not be able to report all of your findings in the abstract. Select approximately two primary results that are most salient to your manuscript. Try to rewrite these sentences so that they are shortened into one to two sentences. Each result should be accompanied by the statistical test result, exact *p* value, and confidence interval.
- Conclusions: Go to your Discussion section and select one to two primary points regarding the implications of your findings for the population and profession. Rewrite these sentences so that they are shortened into one to two sentences.
- Ask a peer who understands research methods to read your abstract and let you know if it is clear, and if not, what can be made clearer.
- If needed, write a second draft and repeat the process of obtaining feedback and making revisions.

Introduction [no heading needed]
The Introduction should be approximately four to five double-spaced, typed pages and should present the background of the problem (as it relates to the population, the profession, and society), the need for the present study, and an analysis of the current related research to date.

Writing Exercises: Introduction

- See the example papers at the end of this chapter to understand how to write clear Introduction sections.

Background [approximately 2–3 paragraphs]
- Practice writing the Introduction section of your manuscript or capstone project.
- Begin by describing the background of the problem as it relates to the clinical population addressed. Most backgrounds begin with information about the prevalence or incidence rate of the addressed clinical condition.

- Describe the current problem with regard to the clinical population's daily life function, community participation, or some other important aspect of their life situation. How have these factors impacted the addressed clinical population?
- Then describe how this problem has impacted the larger society and the profession.

Need for Study [commonly 2 paragraphs]

- The need for the study answers the questions, "Why is this study needed now to help the addressed clinical population?" "How will this study contribute to the knowledge needed to inform clinical practice to assist this population?" For a general research study, the need for the study often addresses the obtaining of knowledge that has not yet been uncovered or investigated.
- Ask a peer who understands research methods to read your Introduction and describe the background and need for your study. If they could not adequately describe the background and need as you intended, identify what they missed and rewrite those components.
- Write a second draft and repeat the process of obtaining feedback and making revisions.

Literature Review

Sometimes a brief review of the current related literature is embedded in the Introduction and is not separately labeled as "Literature Review." In capstone projects and some journals, the Literature Review is labeled with a separate heading, either within the Introduction or as a new section following the Introduction.

The review of related literature should be concisely summarized and highlight key studies and findings. Articles reviewed should have been published within the last 7 years. Classic studies published more than 7 years ago can be reviewed and are the exception to the 7-year rule. If literature published in the last 7 years is lacking, authors should clearly identify this insufficiency. After concisely reviewing the literature, authors should help readers understand the gaps existing in the current literature and the need for the present study. See Chapter 3 for a more in-depth examination explaining the elements of various types of literature reviews.

Writing Exercises: Literature Review [commonly 2–3 double-spaced, typed pages]

- See Chapter 3 for more details about writing different types of literature reviews.
- Begin by reading the example papers at the end of the chapter to gain a clearer understanding of how to write literature reviews.

- Then go to the literature and complete a database search on your topic using key words. Identify all studies within a specified time period that directly relate to your topic.
- The literature review should synthesize the current published information regarding your topic so that readers can gain an understanding of what research has been completed to date.
- Generally, a synthesis means that you will summarize the existing literature using larger categories such as research design, specific population, sample size, findings, and limitations. It may be helpful for you to make a chart to organize this data so that you can present it in narrative form.
- When only a handful (≤5) of studies exist, authors may present more specific information about each of these studies instead of synthesizing them as a group.
- Literature reviews should end with a paragraph about what information is missing from the existing literature and how your study intends to fill this gap in the profession's knowledge base.
- Ask a peer who understands research methods and is familiar with your topic to read your literature review and provide feedback about its exhaustiveness and clarity.
- Make revisions based on the provided feedback.

Final Paragraph before Method [no heading needed]

The purpose statement is the final paragraph of the Introduction, before the Method section begins. Here, authors state the purpose of the present study, and research questions or hypotheses are clearly and explicitly stated. Research questions for a general research manuscript should contain the population, independent and dependent variables, and/or the topical issue examined.

Examples of good research questions include the following:

- What is the relationship between sensory processing disorders and food refusal in children with autism spectrum disorders?
- Do adolescents who are at risk for school failure demonstrate differences in cognitive problem-solving strategies compared to academically successful adolescents?
- What are the perceptions of five homeless adults who received occupational therapy services to transition from a shelter to supportive housing?

Writing Exercises: Purpose Statement

- See the example papers at the end of this chapter for a clearer understanding of how to write a purpose statement.
- Then practice writing a purpose statement for your manuscript or capstone project.
- Begin with "The purpose of this study was to ..." and complete the sentence with the primary objective of your study.

- Example: "The purpose of the present study was to explore the experience of older adults who participated in a driver retraining program after stroke."
- Remember that all research reports and capstone projects are written in the past tense. Research and capstone proposals are written in future tense.

Writing Exercises: Research Questions

- See the example papers at the end of this chapter for a clearer understanding of how to write research questions.
- Practice writing research questions for your study using the guidelines above.
- Make sure to include the population, independent and dependent variables, and/or the topical issue examined.
- Ask a peer to read your research questions and then explain what you are seeking through your study. If the reader is accurate, you have likely written good research questions. If they are not accurate, you may need to revise your research questions based on the labeling strategies outlined above.

Definitions

In the Introduction and throughout the text, authors should define all new and unfamiliar terms for readers as soon as the term is presented. Many authors make the common mistakes of failing to define terms, unclearly defining terms, presenting terms early in the paper and defining them in later sections, or changing the definitions of terms in a paper. There is a formula for writing good definitions. Unless a term is technically defined in the health care community using precise language that could significantly alter the term's meaning if changed, definitions should not be quoted from another source. Instead, all definitions should either be created by the authors or paraphrased and cited.

Good definitions contain the following three elements (Mosey, 1996):

1. Label: The label is the term used to describe a specific concept. The label chosen should be used consistently throughout the paper and should not change.
2. Superordinate concept: The superordinate concept is the larger umbrella term or category under which the term falls.
3. Distinguishing characteristics: Distinguishing characteristics are the concepts that differentiate the term from similar concepts.

Examples of good definitions include the following:

- Repetitive strain disorders are overuse syndromes in which the soft tissues of a joint become inflamed as a result of repeated engagement in activities that require continued movement.

Repetitive strain disorders [label] are overuse syndromes [superordinate concept] in which the soft tissues of a joint become inflamed as a result of repeated engagement in activities that require continued movement [distinguishing characteristics].

- Cognitive problem-solving strategies are executive functions mediated by the frontal lobe that require the ability to identify a problem, plan a strategy, execute the strategy, evaluate the strategy's effect, and modify the strategy as needed.
  Cognitive problem-solving strategies [label] are executive functions mediated by the frontal lobe [superordinate concept] that require the ability to identify a problem, plan a strategy, execute the strategy, evaluate the strategy's effect, and modify the strategy as needed [distinguishing characteristics].
- Food refusal is the rejection of specific food types based on tastes, textures, consistencies, scents, and appearances that are aversive to the child.
  Food refusal [label] is the rejection of specific food types [superordinate concept] based on tastes, textures, consistencies, scents, and appearances that are aversive to the child [distinguishing characteristics].

Writing Exercises: Definitions

- Make sure that all new and unfamiliar terms for readers are defined in your manuscript or capstone project when they first appear. If you are unsure of which terms may be new or unfamiliar to readers, ask a peer to read your work and identify such terms.
- Practice writing good definitions using the guidelines above and ensuring that you have a label, superordinate category, and distinguishing characteristics for all new and unfamiliar terms.
- To practice, define the term "occupational therapy."
- Occupational therapy [label] is a health care profession [superordinate category] that assists people to restore or newly gain participation in desired daily life activities in home and community settings through skilled services, remediation, adaptation, and compensation [distinguishing characteristics].
- After writing several definitions, ask a peer to read them and let you know if they are clear. If they are not clear, ask the reader why or what part of the definition is unclear.
- Then revise the definitions with that feedback. Continue to use labels, superordinate categories, and distinguishing characteristics to structure your revised definitions.

Quotations

In scholarly writing in the health sciences, quotations should only be used to quote a historical or legal document, a technical definition that has been accepted by the scientific community and whose meaning may significantly change if the exact wording is altered, or a specific participant response in a qualitative study. With the exception of the previous instances, quotations should not be used. Instead, paraphrase content and cite the source.

Method

The Method section provides a blueprint of your study procedures so that others can replicate your findings. Using the subheadings listed below to structure your Method section will ensure that you report critical and essential information needed by editors, reviewers, and readers to evaluate the quality of your methods and assess how adequately such methods addressed your study's research questions.

Research Design

Research Design should be the first subheading of the Method section because this information is needed by the reader to understand which study design has been used and whether it can adequately answer the research question. If the research design does not match the study question, the study will be flawed. When the specific research design is not clearly stated in its own section or is embedded within another section, readers must search for this essential information. The research design should be clearly stated and described in several sentences. At the end of this subsection, authors should state that the study was approved (or exempted) by an institutional review board (or ethics committee). Authors should also state that adult participants or guardians provided consent (and that children provided assent).

Writing Exercises: Research Design [approximately 1 paragraph]

- See the example papers listed at the end of this chapter for a clearer understanding of how to write the Research Design subsection.
- Use the checklist at the end of this chapter to make an outline of your Research Design section.
- Write the Research Design section of your Methods, making sure to
  - Thoroughly describe the study's research design.
  - Indicate that either institutional review board or ethics committee approval (or exemption) was obtained.
  - State that informed consent was attained from adult participants or assent from child participants (or both when appropriate).
- Ask a peer who understands research methods to read your Research Design section and let you know if it is clear and contains all needed information. Make revisions as needed.

Participants

Participants is the second subheading in the Methods section. The term *participants*, as opposed to *subjects*, is used in health care research to imply that those selected to participate in the study have willingly volunteered and are actively engaged in the research project. *Subjects* implies that those selected may or may not know that they are in a study and are manipulated by the researcher instead of actively participating in the research process. The term *participants* should be used consistently throughout the text.

In this subsection, authors should concisely describe the recruitment process and inclusion/exclusion criteria for study enrollment. The recruitment process description should specifically address how participants were selected (e.g., from convenience sampling or randomization), by whom, and from what setting. Both inclusion and exclusion criteria for participant selection should be explicitly stated.

Participant demographics, participant flow, and final sample size should not be addressed in this subsection; instead, this information should be provided at the beginning of the Results section.

Writing Exercises: Participants [approximately 1–2 paragraphs]

- See the example papers listed at the end of this chapter to gain a clearer understanding of how to write the Participants subsection.
- Use the checklist at the end of this chapter to make an outline of your Participants section.
- Write the Participants section of your Methods, making sure to
  - Describe how participants were recruited and the sampling methods that were used to select them.
  - State who completed recruitment and describe the setting(s) from which participants were recruited.
  - Provide the precise inclusion/exclusion criteria for participant selection.
- Ask a peer who understands research methods to read your Participants section and describe who your targeted sample was, what sampling method was used to recruit your sample, from what setting(s) participants were recruited, and what were the inclusion/exclusion criteria.
- If your reader could easily identify these, you have likely written a strong Participants section. If they could not, revise your Participants section using the above guidelines. Repeat the process of obtaining feedback and making revisions.

Instruments

The third subheading in the Methods section is Instruments. All instruments used to measure outcomes or dependent variables should be cited and addressed with regard to intended purpose, population for which the instrument was designed and assessed, type of data collected (e.g., self-report, performance-based observer rating, Likert scale, open-ended questions, total score yielding ratio data), and administration length. An instrument's psychometric properties should be reported in numerical value with statistical test results, exact p values, and confidence intervals indicated. All psychometric properties should be cited. If no psychometric properties have been established, or if the instrument was developed specifically for the present study, the authors should state this clearly in the Instruments section rather than addressing these conditions only in the Limitations subsection of the Discussion section. It is often helpful to readers to provide sample item questions in a table or figure when an instrument has been developed by the authors specifically for the present study. For capstone projects, the full instrument can be placed in a figure or appendix at the end of the manuscript.

Writing Exercises: Instruments [approximately 1–3 paragraphs]

- See the example papers listed at the end of this chapter to gain a clearer understanding of how to write the Instruments subsection.
- Then use the checklist at the end of this chapter to make an outline of your Instruments section.
- Using your outline, write the Instruments section of your Methods, making sure to
  - Describe all instruments used to measure study outcomes with regard to
    - Intended purpose
    - Population for which the instrument was designed and assessed
    - Type of data collected
    - Length of administration
  - Provide the citation(s) for all instruments
  - Report the reliability and validity of all instruments. Provide numeric values, statistical tests, exact *p* values, and confidence intervals. Provide citations for reliability and validity data.
  - If an instrument was developed for the present study, this must be explicitly stated. Describe the instrument development process and provide sample items in a table or figure. The full instrument can be placed in a figure or appendix at the end of the manuscript for capstone projects.
- Ask a peer who understands research methods to read your Instruments section and let you know if they understand each instrument's purpose, intended population, type of data that can be collected, administration length, and reliability and validity. If the reader cannot, ask what is unclear and use that feedback to revise your work. Repeat the process of obtaining feedback and making revisions.

Procedures

The Procedures subsection commonly follows the Instruments subsection. Here, authors should report the steps of the study in sufficient detail so that the study can be replicated and so that editors, reviewers, and readers can evaluate it. Procedures should begin with steps that occurred once the study commenced. Recruitment and consent procedures should not be reported here; this information should be addressed in the Research Design and Participants subsections. To promote transparency, authors should report which researcher was responsible for and executed each specific procedure. Authors must clearly report whether researchers and participants were anonymized to participant group assignment and study purpose because these conditions may significantly bias results.

Writing Exercises: Procedures [approximately 3-4 paragraphs]

- See the example papers listed at the end of this chapter to gain a clearer understanding of how to write the Procedures subsection.
- Then use the checklist at the end of this chapter to make an outline of your Procedures section.
- Using your outline, write the Procedures section of your Methods, making sure to
  - Report the steps of the study in sufficient detail so that it can be evaluated and replicated by readers.
  - Do not report recruitment and consent procedures here. Begin the Procedures with the steps that occurred once recruitment and consent were completed.
  - Indicate who was responsible for and implemented each procedural step.
  - Indicate whether researchers and participants were anonymized to participant group assignment and study purpose.
- Ask a peer who understands research methods to read your procedures section and describe it back to you, indicating what is clear and what needs greater clarification. Make revisions based on this feedback. Repeat the process of obtaining feedback and making revisions.

Data Collection

The Data Collection subsection commonly follows the Procedures subsection. The data collection schedule should be clearly reported here—describe how, when, and by whom each set of data was collected. Training procedures for data collectors should be documented, and if multiple data collectors were used, authors should report interrater reliability scores. Authors must also state whether data collectors were anonymized to participant group assignment and whether they were different members of the research team than those who had other roles (such as participant recruiter and participant group allocator). All of this information must be provided so that editors, reviewers, and readers can evaluate whether compromised data collection procedures may have biased results. If any of the above procedures were not addressed in the study, such omissions should be disclosed in the Data Collection subsection rather than discussed only in the Limitations subsection.

Writing Exercises: Data Collection [approximately 2–3 paragraphs]

- See the example papers at the end of this chapter for a clearer understanding of how to write the Data Collection subsection.
- Then use the checklist at the end of this chapter to make an outline of the main points in your Data Collection section.
- Write the Data Collection section of your Methods, making sure to

    - Report the data collection schedule describing how, when, and by whom each set of data was collected.
    - Report the training procedures for data collectors. When multiple data collectors were used, provide interrater reliability scores attained during training.
    - State whether data collectors were anonymized to participant group assignment.
    - Indicate whether data collectors were distinct research team members and separate from those who performed other roles such as recruitment and participant group allocator.
- Ask a peer who understands research methods to read your Data Collection section and describe it back to you, indicating what is clear and what needs greater clarification. Make revisions based on that feedback. Repeat the process of obtaining feedback and making revisions.

Data Analysis

The final subsection of the Methods section is Data Analysis. Here, authors should describe and cite all statistical tests and qualitative methods used to analyze data. The use of nontraditional statistical procedures that are not congruent with traditional parametric and nonparametric data analysis should be justified and cited. Similarly, the use of statistical and qualitative analytic methods that are congruent with established norms but are not familiar to most readers should be described and cited. Authors should indicate which software program was used for statistical or qualitative data analysis, and for quantitative studies, at what significance level probability was set.

Writing Exercises: Data Analysis [approximately 2–3 paragraphs]

- See the example papers at the end of this chapter for a clearer understanding of how to write the Data Analysis subsection.
- Then use the checklist at the end of this chapter to make an outline of the main points in your Data Analysis section.
- Write the Data Analysis section of your Methods, making sure to
    - Describe and cite all statistical tests and qualitative methods used to analyze data.
    - Justify and cite the use of nontraditional statistical procedures that differ from traditional parametric and nonparametric data analysis procedures.
    - Identify and cite the software program used for statistical and qualitative analysis.
    - For quantitative studies, state at what level statistical probability was set.
- Ask a peer who understands research methods to read your Data Analysis section and describe it back to you, indicating what is clear and what needs greater clarification. Make revisions based on that feedback. Repeat the process of obtaining feedback and making revisions.

A concisely written Method section that provides all of the essential information previously listed should consist of approximately five double-spaced, typed pages.

Results

The Results section begins after the end of the Data Analysis subsection of the Method section and commences a new section of the manuscript. In the Results section, you will report your findings without interpreting them; interpretation of findings will be made in the Discussion section. The objective of the Results section is to report your findings in a concise, clear, and sufficient way so that readers can verify reported results. Although it is not customary to provide participant raw scores, authors are increasingly providing this information through online repositories. It is important to report the results in absolute numbers rather than percentages. When percentages are given, they should be accompanied by the absolute numbers from which percentages were derived.

Begin the Results section with information about participant flow and demographics. Participant flow includes information about the number of participants recruited, the number enrolled in the study, the number of participants who withdrew or whose participation was terminated by the researchers, and the final sample size. Reporting standards require that age, gender, race, ethnicity, education level, socioeconomic level, and topic-specific characteristics such as functional status be provided for all participants. Authors should describe power analyses, sample size estimations, and confidence level estimations that were calculated to ensure that the study sample size was adequate to yield reliable statistical results.

After participant flow and demographic information are provided, the remainder of the Results section should be organized in accordance with the order of research questions outlined in the purpose statement (of the Introduction). Findings should be reported for each research question. Missing data should be acknowledged, and the protocol for handling missing data should be described. In a quantitative study, results should be reported using statistical test values, exact p values, and confidence intervals. Reporting confidence intervals with p-values provides a measure of the effect size and its precision. In a qualitative study, findings should be organized by themes with supporting participant quotations.

See Chapter 10, Reporting Statistical Data in Text and Tables, to understand how to correctly report statistical tests and symbols in the Results section.

A concisely written Results section that provides all of the essential information previously mentioned should consist of approximately two to four double-spaced, typed pages.

Writing Exercises: Results [approximately 2–4 double-spaced, typed pages]

- See the example papers at the end of this chapter for a clearer understanding of how to write the Results section.
- Then use the checklist at the end of this chapter to make an outline of the main points in your Results section.

- In your outline, first include information about participant flow and demographics.
- Then order your research questions in accordance with the order listed in the Introduction. Beneath each question, insert the primary points that you want to include.
- Using your outline, write the Results section, making sure to
  - Begin the Results section with information about participant flow and demographics.
  - Report all findings without interpreting them.
  - Report results in absolute numbers rather than percentages. When percentages are provided, indicate the absolute numbers from which the percentages were derived.
  - Report power analyses, sample size estimations, and confidence level estimations that were calculated to ensure that the sample size was adequate to yield reliable results.
  - Organize the remainder of the Results section in accordance with the order of the research questions outlined in the purpose statement of the introduction.
  - Acknowledge missing data and describe the protocol for handling it.
  - Report all quantitative findings in numerical values with statistical test results, exact *p* values, and confidence intervals.
  - Organize and report qualitative findings by themes with supporting participant quotes.
- Finally, ask a peer who understands research methods to read your Results section and describe it back to you, indicating what is clear and what needs greater clarification. Make revisions based on that feedback. Repeat the process of obtaining feedback and making revisions until the Results section has all needed information and is clear.

Discussion

The Discussion section follows the Results section and begins a new section of the manuscript. While the Results is a reporting of your findings without interpretation, the Discussion provides the opportunity to interpret your findings. Findings, however, should not be repeated from the Results section. For clarity, the Discussion section should be organized in accordance with the order of research questions addressed in the Results section. It is the author's objective to answer each research question based on study findings. Unexpected findings should be explained. Authors should discuss whether findings are novel or support previous work in the literature. It is critical that authors do not overstate the meaning of findings but rather present interpretations neutrally and without qualifiers. Authors should clearly state that interpretations apply only to the study sample and not to the larger population. Readers should be left to make decisions regarding interpretation based on the presented data in the Results section. This initial section of the Discussion section is commonly 3–4 double-spaced, typed pages.

Writing Exercises: Discussion [approximately 3–4 double-spaced, typed pages]

- See the example papers listed at the end of this chapter for a clearer understanding of how to write the Discussion section.
- Then use the checklist at the end of this chapter to make an outline of the main points in your Discussion section.
- Begin by ordering your research questions in accordance with the order of research questions addressed in your Results section. Beneath each question, insert the primary points of the Discussion that you want to include.
- Make sure to
  - Explain and interpret all findings without repeating the results. Why might each finding have occurred?
  - Explain unexpected findings (why might these have occurred?).
  - For each finding, describe whether it is novel or supports previous work in the literature.
  - Be sure that your interpretation of findings is not overstated and relates only to your own study sample. Do not generalize findings from your sample to the larger population.
- Use your outline to write a first draft of your Discussion section.
- Once drafted, ask a peer who understands research methods to read your Discussion section and describe it back to you, indicating what is clear and what needs greater clarification. Make revisions based on that feedback. Repeat the process of obtaining feedback and making revisions.

Limitations

The Limitations subheading is inserted in the Discussion section after the previously mentioned information is addressed. Here, authors acknowledge the study limitations that may have biased the results, including small sample size, lack of control and randomization, compromised anonymization procedures, and the use of assessments without established reliability and validity. Authors should discuss the generalizability of the sample to the larger population and address differences between the target population and the study sample. Limitations of qualitative studies may include findings from small sample sizes that are not transferable to the larger population and compromised methods used to ensure data trustworthiness. The Limitations section is approximately 1–2 paragraphs.

Writing Exercises: Limitations [approximately 1–2 paragraphs]

- See the example papers listed at the end of this chapter for a clearer understanding of how to write the Limitations subsection of the Discussion section.
- Then use the checklist at the end of this chapter to make an outline of the main points in your Limitations section.

- Write a first draft of the Limitations section, making sure to
  - Acknowledge all possible limitations that may have biased study results.
  - Describe differences between the target population and the study sample; discuss how these may have impacted the generalizability of findings.
- Ask a peer who understands research methods to read your Limitations section and describe it back to you, indicating what is clear and what needs greater clarification. Make revisions based on that feedback. Repeat the process of obtaining feedback and making revisions.

Future Research

The Future Research subheading is inserted after the Limitations section and is part of the Discussion. Here authors should indicate how future research can address the present study's limitations. Authors can also identify research questions that remain unanswered and suggest directions for future studies. The Future Research section is approximately one to two paragraphs.

Writing Exercises: Future Research [approximately 1–2 paragraphs]

- See the example papers listed at the end of this chapter for a clearer understanding of how to write the Future Research subsection of the Discussion section.
- Then use the checklist at the end of this chapter to make an outline of the main points in your Future Research section.
- Write a first draft of the Future Research section, making sure to
  - Describe how future research can address the study's limitations.
  - Identify research questions that remain unanswered and suggest directions for future studies.
- Ask a peer who understands research methods to read your Future Research section and describe it back to you, indicating what is clear and what needs greater clarification. Make revisions based on that feedback. Repeat the process of obtaining feedback and making revisions.

Implications for Practice

Implications for Practice is also part of the Discussion section and is inserted after Future Research. Here, authors should state how their findings can be used to inform clinical practice. The format for the Implications for Practice section is commonly presented as a narrative paragraph or bulleted list. This section is relatively short at approximately one paragraph or six bullets. The shortness of this section is a recognition that study findings have been derived from one sample that cannot be generalized to the larger population and that further research must be conducted to add to the body of knowledge regarding the topic area.

Writing Exercises: Implications for Practice [approximately 1 paragraph or 6 bullets]

- See the example papers listed at the end of this chapter for a clearer understanding of how to write the Implications for Practice subsection of the Discussion.
- Then use the checklist at the end of this chapter to make an outline of the main points in your Implications for Practice section.
- Write a first draft of the Implications for Practice section, making sure to cautiously suggest how study findings may be used to inform clinical practice.
- Ask a peer who understands research methods to read your Implications for Practice section and describe it back to you, indicating what is clear and what needs greater clarification. Ask the reader to comment on whether you may have overstated your findings' application to practice. Make revisions based on that feedback. Repeat the process of obtaining feedback and making revisions.

Conclusion

The Conclusion is the final subheading of the Discussion section. This section should summarize the study's primary findings and their possible application to practice. A concise, well-written Conclusion section should be approximately 250–300 words.

Writing Exercises: Conclusion [approximately 1–2 paragraphs]

- See the example papers listed at the end of this chapter for a clearer understanding of how to write the Conclusion subsection.
- Then use the checklist at the end of this chapter to make an outline of the main points in your Conclusion section.
- Write a first draft of the Conclusion section, making sure to
  - Summarize the study's primary findings, possible application to clinical practice, and needed future research.
  - Make sure not to overstate study findings.
- Ask a peer who understands research methods to read your Conclusion section and describe it back to you, indicating what is clear and what needs greater clarification.
- Ask the reader to comment on whether you may have overstated your findings or their application to practice. Make revisions based on that feedback. Repeat the process of obtaining feedback and making revisions.

After the Conclusion, the remaining manuscript sections in the order in which they should be presented are as follows:

- References
- Tables
- Figures

Checklist for Manuscript Structure and Content of General Research Studies

Title

- ☐ Include the population, independent variable, dependent variable, and research design.
- ☐ In a professional issue manuscript, include the topical issue in the title.

Abstract

- ☐ Objectives: In one to two sentences, describe the purpose of the study.
- ☐ Method: In one to two sentences, provide information about participants (e.g., population, sample size, recruitment strategies), research design, and data collection procedures.
- ☐ Results: In one to two sentences, report the primary findings along with statistical test results, exact *p* values, and confidence intervals.
- ☐ Conclusions: In one to two sentences, describe the implications of the study for the population and profession.

Introduction [no heading is needed]

- ☐ Present the background of the problem as it relates to the population, profession, and society.
- ☐ Present the need for the present study.

Literature Review [presented as either a separate section or embedded within the Introduction]

- ☐ Present an analysis of the current related literature to date.
- ☐ Help readers understand the gaps existing in the literature that warrant the need for the present study.

Final Paragraph of Introduction [no heading is needed]

- ☐ Purpose statement: State the purpose of the present study.
- ☐ Provide primary and secondary research questions or hypotheses.
- ☐ Make sure that all terms are well defined as soon as they are presented in the manuscript.

Method

Research Design

- ☐ Describe the research design.
- ☐ State that institutional review board or ethics committee approval was obtained.
- ☐ State that participant consent was obtained (when children are participants, their parents/guardians provide consent and children provide assent).

Participants

- ☐ Describe the recruitment process and the sampling methods through which participants were selected.
- ☐ State who completed recruitment and from what settings participants were recruited.
- ☐ Provide inclusion and exclusion criteria for participant selection.

Instruments

- ☐ Describe and cite all instruments used to measure outcomes. Describe the intended purpose, the population for which the instrument was designed and assessed, the type of data collected (e.g., self-report, performance-based observer rating, Likert scale, open-ended questions, total score yielding ratio data), and the administration length.
- ☐ Report and cite the reliability and validity for all instruments in numeric values with statistical test results, exact p values, and confidence intervals.
- ☐ Indicate whether the instrument was developed for the present study, and if so, describe the development process and provide sample items in a table or figure if possible. In capstone projects, the full instrument can be provided in a figure or appendix at the end of the paper.

Procedures

- ☐ Report the steps of the study in sufficient detail so that the study can be evaluated and replicated by readers.
- ☐ Procedures should begin with steps that occurred once recruitment and consent procedures were completed.
- ☐ Report which researcher was responsible for and carried out each specific procedure.
- ☐ Report whether researchers and participants were anonymized to participant group assignment and study purpose.

Data Collection

- ☐ Report the data collection schedule: describe how, when, and by whom each set of data was collected.
- ☐ Document the training procedures for data collectors; if multiple data collectors were used, report interrater reliability scores.
- ☐ State whether data collectors were anonymized to participant group assignment.
- ☐ State whether data collectors were different from other members of the research team than those performing other roles (such as participant recruiter and participant group allocator).

Data Analysis

- ☐ Describe and cite all statistical tests and qualitative methods used to analyze data.
- ☐ Justify and cite the use of nontraditional statistical procedures that are not congruent with traditional parametric and nonparametric data analysis.
- ☐ Describe and cite the use of statistical and qualitative analytic methods that are congruent with established norms but are not familiar to most readers.
- ☐ Identify the software program used for statistical or qualitative analysis.
- ☐ For quantitative studies, state at what significance level probability was set.

Results

- ☐ Report all findings without interpreting them.
- ☐ Report results in absolute numbers rather than percentages; when percentages are provided, also indicate the absolute numbers from which percentages were derived.
- ☐ Begin the Results section with information about participant flow and demographics.
- ☐ Describe power analyses, sample size estimations, and confidence level estimations that were calculated to ensure that the study sample size was adequate to yield reliable statistical results.
- ☐ Organize the remainder of the Results section in accordance with the order of research questions outlined in the purpose statement (of the Introduction).
- ☐ Report findings for each research question.
- ☐ Acknowledge missing data and describe the protocol for handling it.
- ☐ Report quantitative findings in numerical values, with statistical test results, exact p values, and confidence intervals.
- ☐ Organize and report qualitative findings by themes with supporting participant quotations.

Discussion

- ☐ Interpret all findings without repeating the results.
- ☐ Organize the Discussion section according to the order of research questions addressed in the Results section.
- ☐ Explain unexpected findings.
- ☐ Describe whether findings are novel or support previous work in the literature.
- ☐ Be sure that the interpretation of findings relates only to the study sample.

Limitations

- ☐ Acknowledge the study limitations that may have biased the results, including small sample size, lack of control and randomization, compromised anonymization procedures, the use of assessments without established reliability and validity, and compromised methods to ensure trustworthiness of data.
- ☐ Discuss the generalizability of the sample to the larger population and address differences between the target population and the study sample.

Future Research

- ☐ Indicate how future research can address the present study's limitations.
- ☐ Identify research questions that remain unanswered and suggest directions for future studies.

Implications for Practice

- ☐ State how findings may be used to inform clinical practice.

Conclusion

- ☐ Summarize the study's primary findings and their possible application to practice.

Examples of Well-Written General Research Studies

Donica, D. K., Beck, L., & Mumford, K. (2025). Exploring the relationship between handwriting legibility and praxis in third and fourth grade students. *Open Journal of Occupational Therapy, 13*(1), 1–9. https://doi.org/10.15453/2168-6408.2285

Hwang, E. J., Peyton, C. G., Kim, D. K., Nakama-Sato, K. K., & Noble, A. E. (2014). Postdeployment driving stress and related occupational limitations among veterans of Operation Iraqi Freedom and Operation Enduring Freedom. *American Journal of Occupational Therapy*, *68*(4), 386–394. https://doi.org/10.5014/ajot.2014.011668

References

American Psychological Association. (2020). *Publication manual of the American Psychological Association* (7th ed.). Author.

Mosey, A. C. (1996). *Applied scientific inquiry in the health professions: An epistemological orientation* (2nd ed.). American Occupational Therapy Association.

CHAPTER 5

Manuscript Structure and Content for Intervention Effectiveness Studies

The call for evidence-based practice has inspired health care researchers to generate studies evaluating the effect of clinical guidelines. To enhance the quality and transparency of articles describing the methods and results of clinical studies, health care stakeholders have called for the development of reporting standards for intervention studies. This chapter will focus specifically on intervention study reporting standards and the unique information that should be detailed in these types of manuscripts. The information presented next is based on American Psychological Association Guidelines (2020) and the CONSORT Statement (Hopewell et al., 2025) and addresses manuscript structure for clinical research designs, including randomized controlled studies, two-group designs with control (but no randomization), one-group pretest/posttest designs, and single-subject design studies (with several participants). Case reports and case series are described in Chapter 8.

The headings of an intervention effectiveness study manuscript are similar to those of a general research study as described in Chapter 4, and readers are urged to review this section. Using the following headings and addressing the content that belongs in each will help to ensure that you have included essential information sought by editors, reviewers, and readers.

Intervention effectiveness study manuscripts should be approximately 5,000 words in length and 20–25 double-spaced, typed pages. Authors should adhere to the word and page count specifications for intervention effectiveness studies in a selected journal's author guidelines.

Manuscript Headings and Formatting for Intervention Effectiveness Studies

The following heading levels and formatting are based on American Psychological Association guidelines.

DOI: 10.4324/9781003734550-5

Title

Begin the manuscript with a title on a separate title page. The title should be centered, bolded, and typed in uppercase and lowercase letters.

Abstract

The Abstract should be placed on the page directly following the title page. The word *Abstract* should be capitalized, centered, and bolded. If keywords are required, they are inserted directly after the abstract and indented. The term *keywords* is italicized, capitalized, and indented:

Keywords: stroke, community participation, activities of daily living

Introduction

The Introduction begins on the page directly following the abstract. The heading *Introduction* is not typed in the manuscript because the beginning of the manuscript text alerts the reader that the Introduction has begun.

Literature Review

Literature reviews can be (a) embedded within the Introduction without a separate subheading; (b) embedded in the Introduction with a separate subheading that is bolded, capitalized, and flush left; or (c) inserted following the Introduction as a separate section with a heading that is bolded, capitalized, and centered.

Method

The Method section is positioned directly after the Introduction. The heading *Method* is centered, capitalized, and bolded.

Research Design

Research Design is the first subheading in the Method section. It is bolded, capitalized, and flush left.

Participants

Participants is the second subheading in the Method section. It is bolded, capitalized, and flush left.

Instruments

Instruments is the third subheading in the Method section. It is bolded, capitalized, and flush left.

Intervention

Intervention is the fourth subheading in the Method section. It is bolded, capitalized, and flush left.

Intervention Description

Intervention Description is the first subheading of the Intervention subsection. It is flush left, bolded, capitalized, and italicized. The text begins as a new paragraph beneath the subheading.

Interveners

Interveners, or Interventionists, is the second subheading of the Intervention subsection. It is flush left, bolded, capitalized, and italicized. The text begins as a new paragraph beneath the subheading.

Intervention Fidelity

Intervention Fidelity is the third subheading of the Intervention subsection. It is flush left, bolded, capitalized, and italicized. The text begins as a new paragraph beneath the subheading.

Data Collection

Data Collection is the subheading that directly follows Intervention Fidelity. It is bolded, capitalized, and flush left.

Data Analysis

Data Analysis is the subheading that directly follows Data Collection. It is bolded, capitalized, and flush left.

Results

The Results section directly follows Data Analysis and begins a new section of the paper. The heading *Results* is bolded, capitalized, and centered.

Discussion

The Discussion section directly follows the Results and begins a new section of the paper. The heading *Discussion* is bolded, capitalized, and centered.

Limitations

The Limitations subsection is part of the Discussion section but should be highlighted for the reader by a separate subheading within the Discussion section. The subheading *Limitations* is bolded, capitalized, and flush left.

Future Research

The Future Research subsection directly follows the Limitations subsection. This section is also part of the Discussion section and should be highlighted for the reader by a separate subheading label. The subheading *Future Research* is bolded, capitalized, and flush left.

Implications for Practice

Implications for Practice is a subsection of the Discussion section and follows the Future Research section. The subheading *Implications for Practice* is bolded, capitalized, and flush left.

Conclusion

The Conclusion is the final subsection of the Discussion and follows Implications for Practice. The heading is bolded, capitalized, and flush left.

References

References begin on a separate page following the Conclusion. The heading is centered, capitalized, and bolded.

Tables

Tables should be provided after the end of the references and begin on a separate page. Each table should be presented on its own page. Tables are named and presented in accordance with the order in which they are mentioned in the text. The title of the Table is inserted beneath the Table heading:

Table 1 [bolded, capitalized, and flush left]
Participant Demographics [italicized, capitalized, and flush left]

Figures

Figures should be provided after the end of the tables and begin on a separate page. Each figure should be presented on its own page. Figures are named and presented in accordance with the order in which they are mentioned in the text. The title of the Figure is inserted beneath the Figure heading:

Figure 1 [bolded, capitalized, and flush left]
Examples of Participant Quotes [italicized, capitalized, and flush left]

Manuscript Heading Content for Intervention Effectiveness Studies

There should be no repetition of content in the manuscript. The sections and subsections that follow next should not contain overlap and will not if written as suggested.

Title

The title of an intervention study should contain four essential elements to help indexers categorize the article and assist readers to clearly identify the intervention and population addressed.

- Intervention (independent variable)
- Targeted population

- Outcome measures (dependent variable)
- Research design

The acronym PICO is also used to help authors develop good titles:

- P = population
- I = intervention
- C = control or comparison (research design)
- O = outcome measures

Examples of good research titles include the following:

- Effect of a Sensory-Based Social Skill Program for Adolescents with Autism Spectrum Disorder: A Multiple-Baseline, Single-Subject Design
- Effect of a Self-Regulation Intervention for Children With ADHD: A One-Group Pretest/Posttest Design
- Effect of an Educational Community Group for Caregivers of Adult Family Members with Dementia: A Two-Group Controlled Pretest/Posttest Design
- A Comparison of Neurodevelopmental Therapy vs Modified Constraint-Induced Therapy for Adults with Stroke: A Randomized Controlled Trial

Abbreviations in the title should be avoided unless commonly used and understood in the health care community.

Writing Exercises: Abstracts [approximately 150–200 words]

- See the example papers at the end of this chapter to gain a clearer understanding of how to write abstracts.
- The abstract is the last section that should be written after all other manuscript sections are completed.
- Practice writing an abstract for your manuscript using the provided guidelines.
- Objectives: Go to the purpose statement of your manuscript and identify the purpose of the paper. Modify this sentences(s) so that it is not taken verbatim from the manuscript text.
- Method: Go to your Methods section of your manuscript and identify information regarding the following: participants (e.g., population, sample size, recruitment strategy), research design, and data collection procedures. Revise these sentences so that they are not written verbatim and can be shortened and combined into one to two sentences.
- Results: Select the primary findings from your Results section. You will likely not be able to report all of your findings in the abstract. Select approximately two primary results that are most salient to your manuscript. Try to rewrite these sentences so that they are shortened into one to two sentences. Each result should be accompanied by the statistical test result, exact *p* value, and confidence interval.

- Conclusions: Go to your Discussion section and select one to two primary points regarding the implications of your findings for the population and profession. Rewrite these sentences so that they are shortened into one to two sentences.
- Check to ensure that the word count is within the required limitations of the journal to which you are submitting. If needed, go back through all abstract sections and reduce word length.
- Ask a peer who understands research methods to read your abstract and let you know if it is clear, and if not, what can be made clearer.

Writing Exercises: Titles

- Practice writing a title for your intervention effectiveness manuscript using the above guidelines and examples.
- Identify the intervention, population, outcome, and research design and combine these into one title.
- Ask a peer to read your title and tell you what they think your paper is about. If the reader is correct, you have likely written an adequate title. If they are not correct or are confused, you may need to revise your title using the above directions.

Abstract

Similar to a general research manuscript, the abstract of an intervention effectiveness study manuscript is best organized using the following subheadings: (a) objectives, (b) method, (c) results, and (d) conclusions. The content of each subheading, however, differs from that of a general research manuscript with regard to intervention study details. Addressing the specific content of each subheading, as recommended next, will ensure that you provide editors, reviewers, and readers with critical information needed to understand the intervention, targeted population, and research design. Because readers select papers primarily based on abstracts, the provision of this essential information is critical for transparent intervention effectiveness reporting.

- Objectives: In one to two sentences, authors should describe the purpose of the study.
- Method: In one to two sentences, authors should provide information about participants (e.g., population, sample size, recruitment strategy), research design, intervention (for treatment and comparison groups), length of intervention, follow-up points, and outcome measures.
- Results: In one to two sentences, authors should report the primary findings along with statistical test results, p values, effect sizes, and confidence intervals.
- Conclusions: In one to two sentences, authors should (a) describe the implications of their study for the population and profession and (b) address how the findings can be used to inform best practice.

Authors should check a specific journal's author guidelines to determine word count specifications and preferred abstract headings.

Writing Exercises: Abstracts [approximately 150–200 words]

- See the example papers at the end of this chapter to gain a clearer understanding of how to write abstracts.
- The abstract is the last section that should be written after all other manuscript sections are completed.
- Practice writing an abstract for your manuscript using the provided guidelines.
- Objectives: Go to the purpose statement of your manuscript and identify the purpose of the paper. Modify this sentences(s) so that it is not taken verbatim from the manuscript text.
- Method: Go to your Methods section of your manuscript and identify information regarding the following: participants (e.g., population, sample size, recruitment strategy), research design, and data collection procedures. Revise these sentences so that they are not written verbatim and can be shortened and combined into one to two sentences.
- Results: Select the primary findings from your Results section. You will likely not be able to report all of your findings in the abstract. Select approximately two primary results that are most salient to your manuscript. Try to rewrite these sentences so that they are shortened into one to two sentences. Each result should be accompanied by the statistical test result, exact *p* value, and confidence interval.
- Conclusions: Go to your Discussion section and select one to two primary points regarding the implications of your findings for the population and profession. Rewrite these sentences so that they are shortened into one to two sentences.
- Check to ensure that the word count is within the required limitations of the journal to which you are submitting. If needed, go back through all abstract sections and reduce word length.
- Ask a peer who understands research methods to read your abstract and let you know if it is clear, and if not, what can be made clearer.

Introduction [no heading needed]

The Introduction of an intervention effectiveness study manuscript is similar to that of a general research manuscript with regard to length (four to five double-spaced, typed pages) and the need to address (a) the background of the problem as it relates to the population, profession, and society; (b) the need for the study; and (c) a description of the intervention if it is novel and never or rarely previously used. Because the manuscript addresses the effectiveness of a clinical practice method, however, the Introduction should focus on the intervention as it has been used with the targeted population.

Writing Exercises: Introduction

- See the example papers at the end of this chapter to understand how to write clear Introduction sections.

Background [approximately 2–3 paragraphs]

- Practice writing the Introduction section of your manuscript. Begin by describing the background of the problem as it relates to the clinical population addressed. Most backgrounds begin with information about the prevalence or incidence rate of the addressed clinical condition.
- Describe the current problem with regard to the clinical population's daily life function, community participation, or some other important aspect of their life situation. How have these factors impacted the addressed clinical population?
- Then describe how this problem has impacted the larger society and the profession.

Need for Study [commonly 2 paragraphs]

- The need for the study answers the questions, "Why is this study needed now to help the addressed clinical population?" "How will this study contribute to the knowledge needed to inform clinical practice to help this population?"
- For an intervention effectiveness study, the need for the study will address the assessment of (a) a novel intervention for a specific clinical population that has not been tested, (b) an existing intervention for a specific clinical population that has been insufficiently tested, or (c) an existing intervention for a clinical population or age group that needs to be tested with a different clinical population or age group.
- Once you have drafted the background and need statement, ask a peer who understands research methods to read your work and describe the background and need for your study. If the reader could not adequately describe the background and need as you intended, identify what they missed and rewrite those components.
- Once you have revised the background and need statement, repeat this last step with another peer who understands research methods and is unfamiliar with your study.

Writing Exercises: Description of the Intervention [approximately 1–2 paragraphs]

- When an intervention is novel, authors should provide a description of the intervention, its theoretical base, and proposed methods of delivery.
- See the example papers at the end of this chapter to understand how to write a clear description of the intervention within the Introduction.

- Authors should state that they developed this novel intervention to meet a treatment need that was lacking for a specific clinical population.
- Describe the theoretical bases that were used to develop the intervention.
- Describe the intervention as it is intended to be used with the specific clinical population identified.
- Include a description of the intervention's intended delivery methods (e.g., one-to-one therapy, group therapy, video instruction, virtual reality methods).
- Do not describe details such as overall length of intervention, number of sessions per week, and length of each session, or what is typically referred to as dosage and duration. These details will be placed in the Method section.

Literature Review [either embedded in the Introduction or separated with a new heading]

In many journals, the literature review is embedded within the Introduction. Some journals, however, require the Literature Review to be separated by a new heading. When reviewing the literature for readers, authors should describe the results of previous effectiveness studies (with the target population). Authors should identify existing knowledge gaps regarding the intervention and clearly state how the present study will contribute to the profession's best practice. The 7-year rule applies to intervention effectiveness studies—articles reviewed in the Introduction should have been published within the last 7 years; however, classic studies or theoretical papers that were published more than 7 years ago are the exception to this rule. Because many health care professions are in their early evolution in the building of evidence, intervention studies published within the last 7 years may be lacking or insufficient to make best practice decisions. When this is the case, authors should clearly describe this deficiency in the Introduction.

Writing Exercises: Literature Review [commonly 2–3 double-spaced, typed pages]

- See Chapter 3 for more details about writing different types of literature reviews.
- Begin by reading the example papers at the end of the chapter to gain a clearer understanding of how to write literature reviews.
- Then go to the literature and complete a database search on your intervention using key words. Identify all studies within a specified time period that directly relate to your intervention and target population.
- The literature review should synthesize the current published information regarding the intervention's use with your targeted population so that readers can gain an understanding of what research has been completed to date and what may be lacking.
- Generally, a synthesis means that you will summarize the existing literature using larger categories such as research design, specific population, sample size,

findings, and limitations. It may be helpful for you to make a chart to organize this data so that you can present it in narrative form.
- When only a handful (≤5) of intervention studies exist, authors may present more specific information about each of these studies instead of synthesizing them as a group.
- Literature reviews should end with a paragraph about what information is missing from the existing literature and how your study intends to fill this gap in the profession's knowledge base.
- Ask a peer who understands research methods and is familiar with your topic to read your literature review and provide feedback about its exhaustiveness and clarity.
- Make revisions based on the provided feedback.

Final Paragraph Before Method [no heading needed]

The purpose statement is the final paragraph of the Introduction. Here, authors should state the purpose of the intervention effectiveness study and provide clear and precise research questions. Research questions for an intervention effectiveness study should contain the population, intervention, research design, and outcome measures. Examples of good research questions include the following:

- Can a client-centered, sensory-based, nutritional diet decrease food refusal in five conveniently selected children with autism spectrum disorder (ASD) compared to five conveniently selected children with ASD who received family meals as usual?
- Can a cognitive problem-solving program for 10 randomly selected adolescents at risk for school failure decrease school dropout rates compared to matched controls?
- Can an interactive housing skill DVD program help eight conveniently selected homeless men transition from a shelter into supportive housing and maintain housing at 6-month follow-up compared to a comparison group that did not participate in the program?

Writing Exercises: Purpose Statement

- See the example papers at the end of this chapter for a clearer understanding of how to write a purpose statement.
- Then practice writing a purpose statement for your intervention effectiveness study.
- Begin with "The purpose of this study was to ..." and complete the sentence with the primary objective of your study.
- Example: "The purpose of the present study was to assess the effectiveness of a lymphedema reduction movement program for women with lymphedema secondary to mastectomy."
- Remember that all research reports are written in the past tense. Only research proposals are written in future tense.

Writing Exercises: Research Questions

- See the example papers at the end of this chapter for a clearer understanding of how to write research questions.
- Practice writing research questions for your study using the guidelines above.
- Make sure to include the clinical population, intervention (independent variable), research design, and outcome measures (dependent variable).
- Ask a peer to read your research questions and then explain what you are seeking through your study. If the reader is accurate, you have likely written good research questions. If they are not accurate, you may want to revise your research questions based on the labelling strategies outlined above.

Definitions

All new and unfamiliar terms that are presented in the Introduction (and throughout the text) should be defined when the term first appears in the manuscript. Common mistakes include failing to define terms, unclearly defining terms, presenting terms in one section and defining them in another, and changing the definition of a term in a paper. To understand how to write good definitions, authors should refer to Chapter 4.

Quotations

Quotations should not be used in health science scholarly writing with the exception of the following:

- Quoting historical or legal documents
- Quoting a technical definition that has been accepted by the scientific community and whose meaning may significantly change if the exact wording is altered
- Quoting a participant's response in a qualitative study

With the exception of the above instances, quotations should not be used. Instead, authors should paraphrase content and cite the source.

Method

Providing clear, detailed, and precise methods is critical for (a) editors, reviewers, and readers to evaluate a study's internal and external validity; (b) researchers to replicate findings under similar conditions; and (c) practitioners to understand whether an intervention can be applied to their own clients and clinical setting. Transparency in reporting is essential to understand whether an intervention demonstrates effectiveness with a specific clinical population and whether findings can be generalized beyond the study sample. If authors do not provide the essential information to determine the above, manuscripts cannot be evaluated and are often rejected. The use of the following subheadings in the Method section, and the content belonging in each subheading, will help you to provide critical information that editors, reviewers, and readers seek.

Research Design

The Method section of intervention effectiveness manuscripts should begin with a subheading labeled *Research Design*. Detailing the design is critical for readers to understand whether the design can truly answer the research questions and address effectiveness. When authors do not describe the research design or embed it in another section, it is difficult for editors and reviewers to evaluate the study. The type of design should be explicitly labeled (e.g., randomized controlled trial, two-group pretest/posttest with control, one-group pretest/posttest, single-subject design, crossover design, or factorial design). The description of the design should include the number and type of participant groups (treatment and comparison), whether control or randomization was used, when measurements were administered, and whether follow-up data collection measures were used. Authors should state that institutional review board (or ethics committee) approval was obtained (or exempted) and that participant/guardian consent was attained. If children served as participants, authors should indicate whether parental or guardian consent was obtained and whether children provided assent. Authors should additionally state that clinical trial registration was obtained and provide the trial registry name, date of registration, and identifying trial registry number.

Writing Exercises: Research Design [approximately 1 paragraph]

- See the example papers listed at the end of this chapter for a clearer understanding of how to write the Research Design subsection for intervention effectiveness studies.
- Use the checklist at the end of this chapter to make an outline of your Research Design section.
- Write the Research Design section of your Methods, making sure to
  - Thoroughly describe the study's research design.
  - Indicate that either institutional review board or ethics committee approval (or exemption) was obtained.
  - State that informed consent was attained from adult participants or assent from child participants (or both when appropriate).
- Ask a peer who understands research methods to read your Research Design section and let you know if it is clear and contains all needed information.

Participants

The Participants subsection specifically addresses recruitment procedures and inclusion and exclusion criteria. Authors should explicitly state the type of sampling method used to recruit participants (e.g., convenience or randomization), who recruited participants, and from what setting. If randomization was used, authors should specify the method through which the random sequence assignment was generated, whether the recruiter was anonymized to the random assignment process, and whether the researcher who created the random assignment process was different from the researcher who enrolled and assigned participants to groups. All of these methods serve to reduce potential sampling bias. Similarly, if nonrandomized comparison groups or matching was used, authors should describe what method was used to assign participants to group conditions or as matched controls.

Inclusion and exclusion criteria should be clearly provided in sufficient detail so that readers can understand who was (and who was not) the targeted participant group, how similarly this group matched the larger population, and whether the targeted participant group was actually recruited and enrolled in the study. The setting(s) from which participants were recruited should be detailed; participants from varying settings may have different demographics and motives for participation that may be otherwise difficult to discern if not specified in this section. The description of the facility type and geographical region should be noted.

Participant demographics, participant flow, and final sample size are part of the results and should be documented in the Results section rather than the Method section.

Writing Exercises: Participants [approximately 1–2 paragraphs]

- See the example papers listed at the end of this chapter to gain a clearer understanding of how to write the Participants subsection.
- Use the checklist at the end of this chapter to make an outline of your Participants section.
- Write the Participants section of your Methods, making sure to
  - Describe how participants were recruited and the sampling methods that were used to select them.
  - State who completed recruitment and describe the setting from which participants were recruited.
  - Provide the precise inclusion/exclusion criteria for participant selection. Remember that exclusion criteria are not the opposite of inclusion criteria. Exclusion criteria indicate who is ineligible for study inclusion and often include such items as
    - Received a prior treatment for the clinical condition that may bias the present study's results
    - May have a comorbid condition that may bias the present study's results
    - Is not a fluent English speaker
- Ask a peer who understands research methods to read your Participants section and describe who your targeted sample was, what sampling method was used to recruit your sample, from what setting(s) participants were recruited, and the inclusion/exclusion criteria.
- If your reader could easily identify these, you have likely written a good Participants section. If they could not, revise your Participants section using the above guidelines. Repeat the process of obtaining feedback and making revisions.

Instruments

Documentation of the instruments through which you measured your outcomes is essential since outcomes provide information about intervention effectiveness. Instruments should be described in detail so that readers can evaluate whether a selected instrument was appropriate to measure a specific outcome. If inappropriate instruments were used to measure specific outcomes, the findings will have no bearing on the intervention's genuine effectiveness. Instruments should be described with regard to purpose, intended population, type of data collected (e.g., self-report, performance-based observer rating, Likert scale, open-ended questions, or total score yielding ratio data), and administration length. The instrument's psychometric properties relating to reliability and validity should be provided in numeric values, with statistical test results, *p* values, and confidence intervals indicated. It is insufficient to state that the instrument's reliability or validity is *high*; readers should be provided with the numeric values of statistical tests so that they can evaluate the instrument themselves. Both the instrument and its psychometric properties should be cited. If psychometric properties for an instrument have not been established, or if an instrument has been newly developed for the present intervention study, the authors should state this information in the Instruments section. Using an instrument without established psychometric properties for an intervention effectiveness study will yield findings that may not be reliable. Authors should justify their decision to use such an instrument in this section. Waiting for the Limitations subsection of the Discussion to disclose this information will appear as though this critical information has been withheld from readers. Similarly, if authors have developed an instrument for the present intervention effectiveness study, they should at minimum describe the development process and disclose whether an attempt was made to establish face or content validity through the evaluation of an expert panel. If space permits, sample items can be illustrated in a table or figure.

Writing Exercises: Instruments [approximately 1–3 paragraphs]

- See the example papers listed at the end of this chapter to gain a clearer understanding of how to write the Instruments subsection.
- Then use the checklist at the end of this chapter to make an outline of your Instruments section.
- Using your outline, write the Instruments section of your Methods, making sure to
  - Describe all instruments used to measure study outcomes with regard to
    - Intended purpose
    - Population for which the instrument was designed and assessed
    - Type of data collected
    - Length of administration
  - Provide the citation(s) for all instruments
  - Report the reliability and validity for all instruments. Provide numeric values for statistical test results along with exact *p* values and confidence intervals. Provide citations for reliability and validity data.
  - If an instrument was developed for the present study, this must be explicitly stated. Describe the instrument development process and provide sample items in a table or figure.

- Ask a peer who understands research methods to read your Instruments section and let you know if they understand each instrument's purpose, intended population, type of data that can be collected, administration length, and reliability and validity. If the reader cannot, ask what is unclear and use that feedback to revise your work.

Intervention

The intervention section is unique to intervention effectiveness studies, case reports, and case series and is divided into three subsections (Intervention Description, Interveners, and Intervention Fidelity) listed below.

Intervention Description

Authors should describe the intervention and state if the intervention was manualized (or based on a written set of guidelines for practice and training that can be accessed by others). Key elements should be provided, addressing the number and length of sessions and the length of intervention over time, the content of each session and whether sessions were delivered individually or in a group, and whether and how the intervention was tailored for specific clients. Authors should also disclose whether clients received any type of simultaneous clinical service that could have influenced results. If a control or comparison group was used, authors should provide the above information for both treatment and control groups.

Writing Exercises: Intervention Description [approximately 1 paragraph]

- See the example papers listed at the end of this chapter to gain a clearer understanding of how to write the Intervention Description subsection.
- Then use the checklist at the end of this chapter to make an outline of your Intervention Description section.
- Using your outline,
  - Describe the intervention
  - Provide information about intervention manualization
  - Provide information about dosage and duration (the number and length of sessions and the length of intervention over time)
  - Provide information about the content of each session and whether sessions were delivered individually or in a group
  - Provide information about whether and how intervention was tailored for specific participants
- Then provide all of the above information for the comparison group(s).
- Once you have a first draft of your Intervention Description section, ask a peer who understands research methods to read it and describe all elements of the intervention to you (for both the intervention and comparison/control groups). If the reader can accurately do so, you have likely written a thorough Intervention Description section.

- Ask the reader if there is anything that is unclear about the descriptions of the intervention and comparison/control groups. Use this information to make revisions and repeat the process of seeking feedback and making revisions.

Interveners

Key information should be provided about the professionals who administered the intervention. Authors should report the type of professional and number of therapists who administered the intervention, the criteria used to select therapists, therapist experience level, the type of training received to administer the intervention, and whether therapists were anonymized to participant group assignment. If a control or comparison group was used, authors should disclose whether the same therapist(s) provided intervention to the treatment and control/comparison group.

Writing Exercises: Interveners [approximately 1 paragraph]

- See the example papers listed at the end of this chapter to gain a clearer understanding of how to write the Interveners subsection.
- Then use the checklist at the end of this chapter to make an outline of your Interveners section.
- Using your outline, report
  - The type of professional and number of therapists who administered the intervention
  - Criteria used to select therapists
  - Therapist experience level
  - Type of training received to administer the intervention
  - Whether therapists were anonymized to participant group assignment
- Then provide all of the above information for the comparison group(s).
- Once you have a first draft of your Interveners section, ask a peer who understands research methods to read it and describe all information about who the interveners were (for both the intervention and comparison groups). If the reader can accurately do so, you have likely written a thorough Intervener section.
- Ask the reader to identify if there is anything that is unclear about the descriptions of the interveners and use this information to make revisions. Repeat the process of seeking feedback and making revisions.

Intervention Fidelity

Intervention fidelity refers to the procedures used to ensure that the intervention was administered in accordance with a written manual, particularly if more than one intervener was used. Authors should describe the procedures used to ensure intervention fidelity and document whether intervention fidelity was measured using an objective instrument. If intervention fidelity was not assessed, authors should explicitly state this here rather than wait for the Limitations section.

Writing Exercises: Intervention Fidelity [approximately 1 paragraph]

- See the example papers listed at the end of this chapter to gain a clearer understanding of how to write the Intervention Fidelity subsection.
- Then use the checklist at the end of this chapter to make an outline of your Intervention Fidelity section.
- Using your outline, report the procedures used to ensure intervention fidelity. For example, was a checklist of all essential intervention elements used by a researcher who observed all interveners periodically throughout the study to ensure that they consistently followed manualized procedures? If interveners drifted from the intervention protocol, did they receive assistance to return to manualized procedures?
- Ask a peer who understands research methods to read your Intervention Fidelity section and describe how you ensured intervention fidelity in your study.
- If the reader is not accurate in their description or identifies unclear intervention fidelity procedures, revise this section based on that feedback and repeat the process of seeking feedback and making revisions.

All of the above information is necessary for readers to replicate the study and understand whether potential bias occurred that could weaken the reliability of results. If any of the above items were not addressed in the study, it is better for authors to disclose such conditions in this section. Waiting to disclose weaknesses in the Limitations section may cause readers to think that key information regarding study design flaws has been withheld.

Data Collection

The Data Collection subsection should detail how, when, and by whom each set of data in the study was collected. Authors should describe the data collection schedule (i.e., when each set of data was collected and by whom), how data collectors were trained to collect data uniformly, whether interrater reliability was established for data collectors if more than one data collector was used, and whether data collectors were anonymized to participant group assignment. It is critical to disclose whether data collectors were different from interveners or if interveners also collected data; the latter condition introduces possible bias that could influence findings regarding the genuine effectiveness of the intervention.

Writing Exercises: Data Collection [approximately 2–3 paragraphs]

- See the example papers at the end of this chapter for a clearer understanding of how to write the Data Collection subsection.
- Then use the checklist at the end of this chapter to make an outline of the main points in your Data Collection section.
- Write the Data Collection section of your Methods, making sure to
  - Report the data collection schedule describing how, when, and by whom each set of data was collected.

  - Report the training procedures for data collectors. When multiple data collectors were used, provide interrater reliability scores attained during training.
  - State whether data collectors were anonymized to participant group assignment.
  - Indicate whether data collectors were distinct research team members and separate from those who performed other roles such as recruitment and participant group allocator.
- Ask a peer who understands research methods to read your Data Collection section and describe it back to you, indicating what is clear and what needs greater clarification. Make revisions based on that feedback.

Data Analysis

In the Data Analysis subsection, authors should detail the statistical procedures that were used to compare pre- and postintervention measures and provide citations for all statistical methods. When statistical methods that are not congruent with traditional parametric and non-parametric rules of data analysis were used, authors should justify the chosen methods and provide citations. Statistical methods that are congruent with traditional data analysis procedures but will likely be unfamiliar to readers should also be justified and cited. Authors should indicate and cite the software program used to generate statistical calculations and report the level at which statistical significance was set. If a randomized or nonrandomized controlled trial was conducted, it is important to report whether intention-to-treat (ITT) analysis was performed (Molero-Calafell et al., 2024). In ITT analysis, all participants enrolled in a study are included in the final data analysis regardless of whether they received treatment and completed the study. ITT analysis mirrors treatment changes and nonadherence that commonly occur in practice and factors these conditions into the analysis of intervention effectiveness. When study noncompleters are removed from final data analysis, bias is introduced in favor of treatment effectiveness. ITT reduces bias and provides a fuller understanding of intervention effectiveness.

Writing Exercises: Data Analysis [approximately 2–3 paragraphs]

- See the example papers at the end of this chapter for a clearer understanding of how to write the Data Analysis subsection.
- Then use the checklist at the end of this chapter to make an outline of the main points in your Data Analysis section.
- Write the Data Analysis section of your Methods, making sure to
  - Describe and cite the statistical procedures that were used to compare pre- and postintervention measures.
  - Justify and cite the use of all statistical methods that are not congruent with traditional parametric and nonparametric rules of data analysis.

- Justify and cite the use of statistical methods that may be unfamiliar to readers.
- Identify and cite the software program used to generate statistical calculations and report the level at which statistical significance was set.
- If a randomized or nonrandomized controlled trial was conducted, report whether ITT analysis was performed.

• Ask a peer who understands research methods to read your Data Analysis section and describe it back to you, indicating what is clear and what needs greater clarification. Make revisions based on that feedback.

The Method section should be approximately five double-spaced, typed pages in length.

Results

The Results section should begin with a description of participant flow, including the number of participants recruited, the number enrolled, the number assigned to each group condition, the number who received follow-up measures, and the number included in the final analysis. In randomized controlled trials and two-group pretest/posttest designs with control, participant flow should be illustrated using a flow chart (Figure 5.1). Authors should indicate whether ITT analysis was performed and clearly state (a) the number of participants who withdrew (or were withdrawn by the researcher) and for what reasons, if known; (b) the number who were lost to follow-up; and (c) the number who did not adhere to intervention recommendations (and for what reasons, if known). All adverse events occurring as a result of the intervention (in both treatment and comparison groups) should be reported.

Authors should report participant demographics with regard to age, gender, race, ethnicity, education level, socioeconomic level, and topic-specific characteristics such as functional level and independent living status. When demographics are reported, absolute numbers should be provided. If percentages are used, the absolute numbers from which the percentages were derived should be provided. If any of the above-noted demographics were not collected, authors should disclose this.

When reporting the sample size, authors should indicate whether a power analysis was performed to estimate the minimum sample size needed to avoid a Type II error (or an error in which the intervention is believed to be ineffective when in fact it is effective).

After reporting participant flow and demographics, authors should provide information about the equivalence of control/comparison and intervention groups (when comparison or control is used). Procedures used to establish whether control and intervention groups were statistically equivalent on baseline measures should be described. If statistically significant differences exist between the control and intervention groups at baseline, authors should detail the statistical methods used to control or remove differences.

When comparison or control groups are used, authors should report between-group outcomes first. If between-group outcome measures are not statistically significant, it is difficult to justify intervention effectiveness. A common mistake involves the minimization of statistically insignificant between-group differences while highlighting statistically significant within-group findings. In this situation, it is inappropriate to use within-group findings to justify the effectiveness of the intervention when in fact no

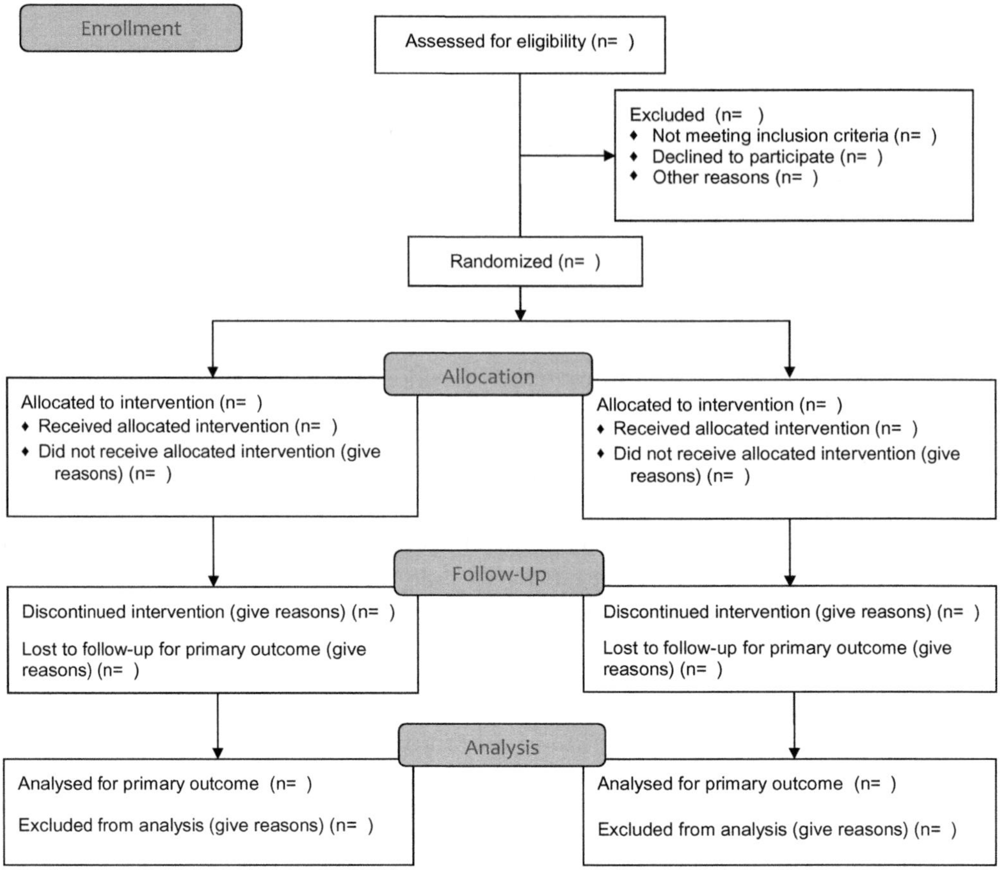

Figure 5.1 Consort Flow Diagram.

Note: Flow diagram of the progress through the phases of a randomized trial of two groups (i.e., enrollment, intervention allocation, follow-up, and data analysis).

Source: Hopewell et al. (2025).

statistically significant differences exist between the intervention group and the control or comparison.

When reporting results, the statistical test value, *p* value, effect size, and confidence intervals should be reported. Effect size allows readers to evaluate whether statistically significant differences between groups (and pre- and posttests) are large enough to be clinically meaningful. Confidence intervals indicate the range of uncertainty for the intervention effect.

Authors should disclose the existence of missing data and describe the statistical methods for handling missing data. Authors should also report whether the intervention was carried out as intended and provide objective data confirming intervention fidelity, if measures were used.

If authors wish to share their raw data in an online repository, this information should be provided either in the Results section or on the title page.

See Chapter 10, Reporting Statistical Data in Text and Tables, to understand how to correctly report statistical tests and symbols in the Results section.

The Results section should be between three and four double-spaced pages in length.

Writing Exercises: Results [approximately 3–4 double spaced, typed pages]

- See the example papers at the end of this chapter for a clearer understanding of how to write the Results section for an intervention effectiveness study.
- Then use the checklist at the end of this chapter to make an outline of the main points in your Data Analysis section.
- In your outline, first include information about participant flow and demographics.
- Then order your research questions in accordance with the order outlined in the Introduction. Beneath each question, insert the primary points that you want to include. Report findings for each research question.
- Using your outline, write the Results section, making sure to
  - Begin with information about participant flow and demographics.
  - In randomized controlled trials and two-group pretest/posttest designs with control, provide a participant flow chart (see Figure 5.1).
  - Indicate whether ITT analysis was performed and provide information about the number of participants who withdrew, were lost to follow-up, and did not adhere to intervention recommendations.
  - Report power analyses, sample size estimations, and confidence level estimations that were calculated to ensure that the sample size was adequate to yield reliable results.
  - Report all findings without interpreting them.
  - Report results using absolute numbers. If percentages are used, also report the absolute numbers from which the percentages were derived.
  - Provide information about the equivalence of intervention and control groups at baseline.
  - Acknowledge missing data and describe the protocol for handling it.
  - Report all quantitative findings in numerical values with statistical test results, exact *p* values, effect size values, and confidence intervals.
  - Report whether intervention was carried out as intended.
  - Report adverse events that occurred as a result of intervention (whether in the intervention or comparison group).
- Finally, ask a peer who understands research methods to read your Results section and describe it back to you, indicating what is clear and what needs greater clarification. Make revisions based on that feedback. Repeat the process of seeking feedback and making revisions.

Discussion

The Discussion section allows authors to interpret their findings for readers. It is critical, however, that authors do not overstate or inflate intervention effectiveness. Findings about the intervention's effectiveness should always be interpreted with caution and the acknowledgement that interpretations can only be applied to the study sample (rather than the larger population). Findings should also be discussed with regard to efficacy and effectiveness. *Efficacy* refers to the effect of an intervention under the tightly controlled conditions of a research setting. *Effectiveness* refers to the effect of an intervention under the practical, real-life conditions of a clinical setting. An intervention that demonstrates efficacy with a specific population under tightly controlled research conditions may not be as potent in a real-life clinical setting in which patient adherence and acceptance, daily time restraints, therapist skill level, and available resources can affect intervention feasibility and outcome.

The Discussion section should be organized in accordance with the order of research questions provided in the purpose statement and addressed in the Results section. Authors should attempt to answer each research question based on findings provided in the Results section. Unanticipated findings should be explained, and authors should discuss whether intervention effectiveness findings are novel or support previous studies. Because several intervention studies are required before consensus can be established regarding intervention effectiveness for a specific population, authors should refrain from suggesting that the intervention in question is effective beyond the study sample unless their research supports a body of already established evidence. If a body of research has not been established, authors should explain how their findings contribute to a growing consensus regarding best practice.

Writing Exercises: Discussion [approximately 3–4 double-spaced, typed pages]

- See the example papers listed at the end of this chapter for a clearer understanding of how to write the Discussion section for an intervention effectiveness study.
- Then use the checklist at the end of this chapter to make an outline of the main points in your Discussion section.
- Begin by ordering your research questions in accordance with the order of research questions addressed in the Results section. Beneath each question, insert the primary points of the Discussion that you want to include.
- Make sure to
  - Explain and interpret all findings without repeating the results. Why might each finding have occurred?
  - Explain unexpected findings (why might these have occurred?).
  - For each finding, describe whether it is novel or supports previous work in the literature.
  - Be sure that your interpretation of findings is not overstated and relates only to your own study sample. Do not generalize findings from your sample to the

larger population. Instead, explain how your findings contribute to a growing consensus regarding best practice.

- Use your outline to write a first draft of your Discussion section.
- Once drafted, ask a peer who understands research methods to read your Discussion section and describe it back to you, indicating what is clear and what needs greater clarification. Make revisions based on that feedback.
- Once you have a second draft, repeat the process of obtaining feedback and making revisions.

Limitations

Confounding variables that may have reduced the study's internal and external validity should be acknowledged. Factors weakening the study's internal validity—the degree to which researchers can be confident that the intervention was responsible for changes in outcome measures—should be addressed. These include lack of intervention fidelity, compromised anonymization procedures of the interveners and/or data collectors, varying therapist skill level, insufficient sample size power, lack of control and/or randomization, and use of assessments having weak or no established psychometric properties. Factors weakening external validity—the degree to which researchers can be confident that the participants represent the larger population—should be detailed. These include compromised anonymization procedures of the group allocator, biased recruitment and enrollment, compromised sampling methods, and the possible influence of participant incentives. A further limitation of many intervention effectiveness studies is a lack of follow-up points, without which researchers cannot understand whether the intervention's effect lasted over time.

Writing Exercises: Limitations [approximately 1–2 paragraphs]

- See the example papers listed at the end of this chapter for a clearer understanding of how to write the Limitations subsection.
- Then use the checklist at the end of this chapter to make an outline of the main points in your Limitations section.
- Write a first draft of the Limitations section of your Discussion making sure to acknowledge factors that may have weakened the study's internal validity, for example:
  - Lack of intervention fidelity
  - Compromised anonymization procedures of the interveners and/or data collectors
  - Varying therapist skill level
  - Insufficient sample size power
  - Lack of control and/or randomization
  - Use of assessments having weak or no established psychometric properties

- Also acknowledge factors that may have weakened the study's external validity, for example:
  - Compromised anonymization procedures of the group allocator
  - Biased recruitment and enrollment procedures
  - Compromised sampling methods
  - The possible influence of participant incentives
- Once you have written a first draft of the Limitations section, ask a peer who understands research methods to read your Limitations section and describe it back to you. Ask the reader to indicate what is clear and what needs greater clarification. Make revisions based on that feedback.
- When you have revised the Limitations into a second draft, repeat the process of obtaining feedback and making revisions.

Future Research

Authors should suggest how future studies can address the present study's limitations and identify which questions regarding intervention use must still be answered. For example, is the intervention cost- and time-efficient? Can patients tolerate the intervention, and if not, how can it be improved? Although the intervention has been found to be effective with children, can it be used with adolescents and adults having the same diagnosis?

Writing Exercises: Future Research [approximately 1–2 paragraphs]

- See the example papers listed at the end of this chapter for a clearer understanding of how to write the Future Research subsection.
- Then use the checklist at the end of this chapter to make an outline of the main points in your Future Research section.
- Write a first draft of the Future Research section of your Discussion, making sure to
  - Describe how future research can address the study's limitations.
  - Identify research questions that remain unanswered and suggest directions for future studies.
- Ask a peer who understands research methods to read your Future Research section and describe it back to you, indicating what is clear and what needs greater clarification. Make revisions based on that feedback.
- Write a second draft and repeat the process of obtaining feedback and making revisions if needed.

Implications for Practice

Authors should cautiously state how their findings may be used to inform clinical practice. The format for the Implications for Practice section is commonly presented as a narrative paragraph or bulleted list. This short section is commonly no more than one paragraph or six bullets. The shortness of this section is a recognition that study findings have been derived from one sample that cannot be generalized to the larger population and that further research must be conducted to add to the body of knowledge regarding the topic area.

Writing Exercises: Implications for Practice [approximately 1 paragraph or six bullets]

- See the example papers listed at the end of this chapter for a clearer understanding of how to write the Implications for Practice subsection.
- Then use the checklist at the end of this chapter to make an outline of the main points in your Implications for Practice section.
- Write a first draft of the Implications for Practice section of your Discussion, making sure to cautiously suggest how study findings may be used to inform clinical practice. Remember that a body of intervention effectiveness research is needed for a specific intervention and clinical population to build consensus for best practice and that your study is just one that is needed to contribute to consensus building.
- Ask a peer who understands research methods to read your Implications for Practice section and describe it back to you, indicating what is clear and what needs greater clarification. Also ask the reader to provide feedback regarding whether your implications for practice are overstated or too far generalized to the larger population. Make revisions based on that feedback.
- If needed, write a second draft and repeat the process of obtaining feedback and making revisions.

Conclusion

In this final section of the manuscript text, authors should summarize the major study findings and describe what these findings mean to the profession, clinical population, and practice.

Writing Exercises: Conclusion [approximately 1–2 paragraphs]

- See the example papers listed at the end of this chapter for a clearer understanding of how to write the Conclusion subsection.
- Then use the checklist at the end of this chapter to make an outline of the main points in your Conclusion section.
- Write the Conclusion section, making sure to
  - Summarize the study's primary findings, possible application to clinical practice, and needed future research.
  - Make sure not to overstate study findings or generalize them to the larger population.
- Ask a peer who understands research methods to read your Conclusion section and describe it back to you, indicating what is clear and what needs greater clarification. Make revisions based on that feedback.
- If needed, write a second draft and repeat the process of obtaining feedback and making revisions.

The Discussion section should be approximately four to five double-spaced, typed pages in length.

After the Conclusion, the remaining manuscript sections in the order in which they should be presented are as follows:

- References
- Tables
- Figures

Checklist for Manuscript Structure and Content of Intervention Effectiveness Studies

Title

☐ Include the following elements: intervention (independent variable), targeted population, outcome measures (dependent variable), and research design (control, comparison).

Abstract

☐ Objectives: In one to two sentences, describe the purpose of the study.

☐ Method: In one to two sentences, provide information about participants (e.g., population, sample size, recruitment strategy), research design, intervention (for treatment and control groups), length of intervention, follow-up points, and outcome measures.

☐ Results: In one to two sentences, report the primary findings along with statistical test results, *p* values, effect sizes, and confidence intervals.

☐ Conclusions: In one to two sentences, (a) describe the implications of the study for the population and profession and (b) address how the findings can be used to inform best practice.

Introduction [no heading needed]

☐ Describe the background of the problem as it relates to the population, profession, and society.

☐ Describe why your study is needed at this time.

☐ For a novel intervention, provide a description of the intervention, its theoretical base, and typical methods of delivery.

Literature Review [presented as either a separate section or embedded within the Introduction]

☐ Describe the intervention's use with the targeted population and the results of previous intervention effectiveness studies with the population.

☐ Identify existing knowledge gaps regarding the intervention and clearly state how the present study will contribute to the profession's best practice.

Final Paragraph of Introduction [no heading is needed]

- ☐ Purpose statement: state the purpose of the intervention effectiveness study.
- ☐ Provide primary and secondary research questions.
- ☐ Make sure that all terms are well defined as soon as they are presented in the manuscript.

Method

Research Design

- ☐ Describe the research design (e.g., randomized controlled trial, two-group pretest/posttest with control, one-group pretest/posttest, single-subject design, crossover design, or factorial design).
- ☐ Include the number and type of participant groups (treatment and control), whether control or randomization was used, when measurements were administered, and whether follow-up data collection measures were used.
- ☐ State that institutional review board (or ethics committee) approval was obtained (or exempted) or that participant or guardian consent was attained. If children served as participants, indicate whether parental or guardian consent was obtained and whether children provided assent.
- ☐ State that clinical trial registration was obtained and provide the trial registry name, date of registration, and identifying trial registry number.

Participants

- ☐ State the type of sampling method used to recruit participants (e.g., convenience, randomization), who recruited participants, and from what setting.
- ☐ If randomization was used, specify the method through which the random sequence assignment was generated, whether the recruiter was anonymized to the random assignment process, and whether the researcher who created the random assignment process was different from the researcher who enrolled and assigned participants to groups.
- ☐ If nonrandomized control groups or matching was used, describe what method was used to assign participants to group conditions or as matched controls.
- ☐ Provide inclusion and exclusion criteria in sufficient detail so that readers can understand who was (and who was not) the targeted participant group, how similarly this group matched the larger population, and whether the targeted participant group was actually recruited and enrolled in the study.
- ☐ If one or more sites were used, describe the facility types and geographical region.

Instruments

- ☐ Describe instruments with regard to purpose, intended population, type of data collected (e.g., self-report, performance-based observer rating, Likert scale, open-ended questions, total score yielding ratio data), and administration length. Cite all instruments.
- ☐ Provide and cite the instrument's psychometric properties in numeric values, with statistical test results, *p* values, and confidence intervals.
- ☐ Justify the use of instruments with little or no established psychometric properties.

- ☐ If an instrument was developed for the present intervention effectiveness study, describe the development process and whether an attempt was made to establish face or content validity through the evaluation of an expert panel. Sample items can be illustrated in a table or figure.

Intervention

Intervention Description

- ☐ Describe the intervention and state whether the intervention is manualized (or based on a written set of guidelines for practice and training that can be accessed by others).
- ☐ Provide information about the number and length of sessions and the length of intervention over time, the content of each session, whether sessions were delivered individually or in a group, and whether and how the intervention was tailored for specific clients.
- ☐ Indicate whether clients received any type of simultaneous clinical service that could have influenced results.
- ☐ Provide all of the above information for both treatment and control/comparison groups (if controls/comparisons were used).

Interveners

- ☐ Report the type of professional and number of therapists who administered the intervention, criteria used to select therapists, therapist experience level, type of training received to administer the intervention, and whether therapists were anonymized to participant group assignment.
- ☐ If a control or comparison group was used, disclose whether the same therapist(s) provided intervention to the treatment and control/comparison groups.

Intervention Fidelity

- ☐ Describe the procedures used to ensure intervention fidelity and document whether intervention fidelity was measured using an objective instrument.
- ☐ Clearly indicate whether intervention fidelity was not addressed.

Data Collection

- ☐ Describe the data collection schedule (i.e., when each set of data was collected in the study and by whom).
- ☐ Describe how data collectors were trained to collect data uniformly and whether interrater reliability was established for data collectors if more than one data collector was used.
- ☐ Describe whether data collectors were anonymized to participant group assignment.
- ☐ Disclose whether data collectors were different from interveners.

Data Analysis

- ☐ Describe and cite the statistical procedures that were used to compare pre- and postintervention measures.
- ☐ Justify and cite the use of statistical methods that are not congruent with traditional parametric and nonparametric rules of data analysis.
- ☐ Justify and cite the use of statistical methods that may be unfamiliar to readers.

- ☐ Indicate and cite the software program used to generate statistical calculations and report the level at which statistical significance was set.
- ☐ If a randomized or nonrandomized controlled trial was conducted, report whether ITT analysis was performed.

Results

- ☐ Begin the Results section with a description of participant flow, including the number of participants recruited, the number enrolled, the number assigned to each group condition, the number who received follow-up measures, and the number included in the final analysis.
- ☐ In randomized controlled trials and two-group pretest/posttest designs with control, illustrate participant flow with a flow chart.
- ☐ Report participant demographics with regard to age, gender, race, ethnicity, education level, socioeconomic level, and topic-specific characteristics such as functional level and independent living status.
- ☐ Indicate whether ITT analysis was performed and clearly state the (a) number of participants who withdrew (or were withdrawn by the researcher) and for what reasons, if known; (b) the number who were lost to follow-up; and (c) the number who did not adhere to intervention recommendations (and for what reasons, if known).
- ☐ Report all adverse events occurring as a result of the intervention (in both treatment and comparison groups).
- ☐ Describe power analyses, sample size estimations, and confidence level estimations that were calculated to ensure that the study sample size was adequate to yield reliable statistical results.
- ☐ Provide information about the equivalence of control and intervention groups at baseline (when comparison or control was used).
- ☐ When reporting results, the statistical test value, p value, effect size, and confidence intervals should be reported.
- ☐ Acknowledge the existence of missing data and describe the statistical methods for handling missing data.
- ☐ Report whether the intervention was carried out as intended and provide objective data confirming intervention fidelity.
- ☐ If appropriate, provide information needed to access the online repository site for data sharing purposes (this information may alternatively be listed on the title page).

Discussion

- ☐ Interpret all findings without repeating the results.
- ☐ Organize the Discussion section according to the order of research questions addressed in the Results section.
- ☐ Explain unexpected findings.
- ☐ Describe whether findings are novel or support previous work in the literature.
- ☐ Be sure that the interpretation of findings relates only to the study sample. Explain how your findings contribute to a growing consensus regarding best practice.

Limitations

- ☐ Acknowledge factors weakening internal validity, for example:
  - ☐ Lack of intervention fidelity, compromised anonymization procedures of the interveners and/or data collectors, varying therapist skill level, insufficient sample size power, lack of control and/or randomization, and use of assessments having weak or no established psychometric properties.
- ☐ Acknowledge factors weakening external validity, for example:
  - ☐ Compromised anonymization procedures of the group allocator, biased recruitment and enrollment, compromised sampling methods, and the possible influence of participant incentives.

Future Research

- ☐ Suggest how future studies can address the present study's limitations and identify which questions regarding intervention use must still be answered.

Implications for Practice

- ☐ Cautiously state how findings may be used to inform clinical practice, making sure not to inflate findings or generalize them beyond the present study sample.

Conclusion

- ☐ Summarize the major study findings and describe what these findings mean to the profession, clinical population, and professional practice.

Examples of Well-Written Intervention Effectiveness Studies

Arnaud, L. M., & Gutman, S. A. (2020). Effectiveness of an occupational therapy reading program for low socioeconomic first and second graders in an urban elementary school: A pilot randomized controlled study. *Journal of Occupational Therapy, Schools, & Early Intervention, 13*(3), 302–319. https://doi.org/10.1080/19411243.2020.1732260

Green, T. M., Fromm, N. M., Gayle, F. S., Lee, J., Wang, W., & Vas, A. K. (2023). Examining the delivery mode of mental practice in reducing hemiparesis: A randomized controlled trial. *Open Journal of Occupational Therapy, 11*(4), 1–9. https://doi.org/10.15453/2168-6408.2149

Gutman, S. A., Balasubramanian, S., Herzog, M., Kim, E., Swirnow, H., Retig, Y., & Wolff, S. (2020). Effectiveness of a tailored intervention for women with ADHD and ADHD symptoms: A randomized controlled study. *American Journal of Occupational Therapy, 74*, 7401205010. https://doi.org/10.5014/ajot.2020.033316

References

American Psychological Association. (2020). *Publication manual of the American Psychological Association* (7th ed.). Author.

Hopewell, S., Chan, A. W., Collins, G. S., Hróbjartsson, A., Moher, D., Schulz, K. F., Tunn, R., Aggarwal, R., Berkwits, M., Berlin, J. A., & Bhandari, N. (2025). CONSORT 2025 statement: Updated guideline for reporting randomised trials. *BMJ, 388*, e081123. https://dx.doi.org/10.1136/bmj-2024-081123

Molero-Calafell, J., Burón, A., Castells, X., & Porta, M. (2024). Intention to treat and per protocol analyses: Differences and similarities. *Journal of Clinical Epidemiology, 173*, 111457. https://doi.org/10.1016/j.jclinepi.2024.111457

CHAPTER 6

Manuscript Structure and Content for Instrument Development and Testing Studies

Instrument development and testing studies hold great significance for a health profession's advancement because intervention effectiveness cannot be demonstrated without reliable and valid assessments. Without studies that establish the psychometric properties of instruments, evidence-based research and practice cannot occur. It is critical that occupational therapists develop reliable and valid instruments that measure the services they render. For example, although occupational therapists help people with disabilities to enhance functional performance in daily occupations and community participation, the profession is in the early stages of developing assessments that measure functional daily activity in the home and community. Such instruments are considered to be ecologically valid and more accurately address the outcomes of occupational therapy practice. When occupational therapists use assessments developed by other professionals that do not address function in the context of real-life activities, reliable information cannot be discerned about the effectiveness of occupational therapy services.

Similar to intervention effectiveness manuscripts, there is a uniform way to report the findings of instrument development and testing studies that promotes transparency and allows readers to assess whether the standards for good methodological quality have been met. This section will focus on the unique content and structure of instrument development and testing study manuscripts and is based on the COSMIN reporting guideline for studies on measurement properties of patient-reported outcome measures (Gagnier et al., 2025).

The length of instrument development and testing study manuscripts varies depending on the number of psychometric properties addressed in the study; however, authors should aim for a length of approximately 5,000 words.

DOI: 10.4324/9781003734550-6

Manuscript Headings and Formatting for Instrument Development and Testing Studies

The following heading levels are based on American Psychological Association (2020) formatting.

Title

Begin the manuscript with a title on a separate title page. The title should be centered, bolded, and typed in uppercase and lowercase letters.

Abstract

The Abstract should be placed on the page directly following the title page. The word *Abstract* should be capitalized, bolded, and centered. If keywords are required, they are inserted directly after the abstract and indented. The term *keywords* is italicized, capitalized, and indented:

Keywords: stroke, community participation, activities of daily living

Introduction

The Introduction begins on the page directly following the abstract. The heading *Introduction* is not typed in the manuscript because the beginning of the manuscript text alerts the reader that the Introduction has begun.

Literature Review

Literature reviews can be (a) embedded within the Introduction without a separate subheading; (b) embedded in the Introduction with a separate subheading that is bolded, capitalized, and flush left; or (c) inserted following the Introduction as a separate section with a heading that is bolded, capitalized, and centered.

Method

The Method section is positioned directly after the Introduction. The heading *Method* is bolded, capitalized, and centered.

Research Design

Research Design is the first subheading in the Method section. It is bolded, capitalized, and flush left.

Participants

Participants is the second subheading in the Method section. It is bolded, capitalized, and flush left.

Instruments

Instruments is the third subheading in the Method section. It is bolded, capitalized, and flush left.

Procedures

Procedures is the fourth subheading in the Method section. It is bolded, capitalized, and flush left.

Data Collection

Data Collection is the subheading that directly follows Procedures. It is bolded, capitalized, and flush left.

Data Analysis

Data Analysis is the subheading that directly follows Data Collection. It is bolded, capitalized, and flush left.

Results

The Results section directly follows Data Analysis and begins a new section of the paper. The heading *Results* is bolded, capitalized, and centered.

Discussion

The Discussion section directly follows the Results and begins a new section of the paper. The heading *Discussion* is bolded, capitalized, and centered.

Limitations

The Limitations subsection is part of the Discussion section but should be highlighted for the reader by a separate subheading within the Discussion section. The subheading *Limitations* is bolded, capitalized, and flush left.

Future Research

The Future Research subsection directly follows the Limitations subsection. It is also part of the Discussion section and should be highlighted for the reader by a separate subheading. The subheading *Future Research* is bolded, capitalized, and flush left.

Implications for Practice

Implications for Practice is a subsection of the Discussion section and follows the Future Research section. The subheading *Implications for Practice* is bolded, capitalized, and flush left.

Conclusion

The Conclusion is the final subsection of the Discussion and follows Implications for Practice. The heading is bolded, capitalized, and flush left.

References

References begin on a separate page following the Conclusion. The heading is centered, capitalized, and bolded.

Tables

Tables should be provided after the end of the references and begin on a separate page. Each table should be presented on its own page. Tables are named and presented in accordance with the order in which they are mentioned in the text. The title of the Table is inserted beneath the Table heading:

Table 1 [bolded, capitalized, and flush left]
Participant Demographics [italicized, capitalized, and flush left]

Figures

Figures should be provided after the end of the tables and begin on a separate page. Each figure should be presented on its own page. Figures are named and presented in accordance with the order in which they are mentioned in the text. The title of the Figure is inserted beneath the Figure heading:

Figure 1 [bolded, capitalized, and flush left]
Interrater Reliability Mean Scores [italicized, capitalized, and flush left]

Manuscript Heading Content for Instrument Development and Testing Studies

There should be no repetition of content in the manuscript. The sections and subsections mentioned next should not contain overlap and will not if written as suggested.

Title

Providing essential elements in the title of an instrument development and testing study will ensure that the study reaches researchers and practitioners interested in the instrument's use.

Titles of instrument studies should contain the following three elements:

1. The population
2. The instrument name or the construct measured
3. The psychometric properties addressed

The following are examples of good titles for instrument development and testing studies:

- Interrater Reliability of the Home Assessment Scale for Elderly with Low Vision
- Content Validity of the Mild Brain Injury Assessment for Children in the Classroom
- Convergent Validity Between Driving Simulators and On-Road Assessments in Adults with Parkinson's Disease

Abbreviations should be avoided unless commonly used and understood in the health care community.

Writing Exercises: Titles

- Practice writing a title for your manuscript using the above guidelines.
- Identify the population, instrument name or the construct measured, and the psychometric properties addressed. Ensure that all of these appear in the title.
- Ask a peer to read your title and describe what they think your paper is about. If they are correct, you have likely written an adequate title. If they are not correct, revise your title using the above directions. Repeat the process of seeking feedback and making revisions.

Abstract

Authors should check a specific journal's author guidelines to determine the formatting requirements for abstracts. Unless specified otherwise, the abstract for instrument development and testing manuscripts should be organized by the following subheadings: (a) objectives, (b) method, (c) results, and (d) conclusions. Using these subheadings—and the content required in each subheading—will ensure that you provide readers with critical information about the instrument, the construct measured, the targeted population, and the quality of the methodology and findings. Most abstracts are between 150 and 200 words; however, authors should check and adhere to the word count specifications outlined in a journal's author guidelines.

- Objectives: In one to two sentences, authors should describe the purpose of the study, which will address the development or further refinement of an instrument and/or the assessment of its psychometric properties.
- Method: In one to two sentences, authors should provide information about the research design, study timeline, participants (population, sample size), and data collection procedures.
- Results: In one to two sentences, authors should report the primary findings along with statistical test results as calculated using either classical test theory (CTT) or item response theory (IRT).
- Conclusions: In one to two sentences, authors should describe the implications of their findings for the instrument's use with the targeted population.

Writing Exercises: Abstracts [approximately 150–200 words]

- See the example papers at the end of this chapter to gain a clearer understanding of how to write abstracts.
- The abstract is the last section that should be written after all other manuscript sections are completed.
- Practice writing an abstract for your manuscript using the above guidelines.
- Objectives: Go to the purpose statement of your manuscript and identify the purpose of the paper. Modify this sentences(s) so that it is not taken verbatim from the manuscript text.

- Method: Go to your Methods section of your manuscript and identify information regarding the following: research design, study timeline, participants (population, sample size), and data collection procedures. Revise these sentences so that they are not written verbatim and can be shortened and combined into one to two sentences.
- Results: Select the primary findings from your Results section. You will likely not be able to report all of your findings in the abstract. Select approximately two primary results that are most salient to your manuscript. Try to rewrite these sentences so that they are shortened into one to two sentences. Each result should be accompanied by the statistical test result, exact *p* value, and confidence interval.
- Conclusions: Go to your Discussion section and select one to two primary points regarding the implications of your findings for the instrument's use with the targeted population. Rewrite these sentences so that they are shortened into one to two sentences.
- Ask a peer who understands research methods to read your abstract and let you know if it is clear, and if not, what can be made clearer.
- If needed, write a second draft and repeat the process of obtaining feedback and making revisions.

Introduction [no heading needed]

The Introduction of an instrument study should describe the background of the problem as it relates to the population, profession, and society (i.e., the need for an instrument that measures a specific construct with a targeted population to enhance evaluation and practice). Information about the incidence of the population for which the instrument has been targeted should be provided with recent citations. The impact of the diagnosis or clinical problem on functional community participation should be discussed so that readers understand the significance of the clinical problem as it relates to the larger society. The construct measured by the instrument should be defined; all novel or unfamiliar terms should also be defined as soon as they are presented in the manuscript (see information about writing good definitions in Chapter 4).

As mentioned earlier, a critical need for the development of many occupational therapy assessments relates to the lack of established instruments having ecological validity, or the ability to measure a patient's functional performance in real-life everyday activities. The need for most instrument studies will address this problem or one of the following situations:

- The instrument has been recently developed and requires the establishment of psychometric properties.
- The psychometric properties of an instrument have been established using CTT but could be strengthened using IRT.
- The instrument has been revised, and psychometric properties must be established for the revision (e.g., a short version of an instrument has been newly developed based on the original long version).

- The instrument was developed in one language, and psychometric properties were established for that version. The instrument has now been translated into another language, and psychometric properties must be established for the translated version.

Writing Exercises: Introduction

- See the example papers at the end of this chapter to understand how to write clear Introduction sections.

Background [approximately 2–3 paragraphs]

- Make an outline of your background using the checklist at the end of this chapter.
- Begin a first draft of your Introduction by describing the background of the problem as it relates to the clinical population addressed.
- The background for an instrument development and testing study commonly addresses the need for an instrument that measures a specific construct with a targeted population to enhance evaluation and practice.
- Most backgrounds begin with information about the prevalence or incidence rate of the addressed clinical condition.
- Describe the impact of the diagnosis or clinical problem on functional community participation.
- Then describe how this problem has impacted the larger society and the profession.

Need for Study [commonly 2 paragraphs]

- The need for the study answers the questions, "Why is this study needed now to help the addressed clinical population?" "How will this study contribute to the knowledge needed to inform clinical practice to assist this population?" For an instrument development and testing study, the need for the study often addresses the need to develop an instrument that can measure functional performance for a specific clinical population and the need to establish psychometric properties for this instrument.
- Make sure to define the construct measured by the instrument, as well as all novel or unfamiliar terms when they are first mentioned in the text.
- Ask a peer who understands research methods to read your Introduction and describe the background and need for your study. If they could not adequately describe the background and need as you intended, identify what they missed and rewrite those components.
- Write a second draft and repeat the process of obtaining feedback and making revisions.

Literature Review

In most instrument development and testing studies, the literature review is embedded in the Introduction and does not have a separate heading. Check the author guidelines of the journal to which you will be submitting to determine if the literature review should be embedded in the Introduction or written as a separate section.

For a newly developed instrument, authors should discuss the literature examining the assessment of the construct with the targeted population through the use of other instruments. The need for the newly developed or revised instrument in the present study should be made clear against the context of previous measures or lack thereof. Authors should briefly describe the instrument (a detailed description of the instrument will be made in the Method section).

Writing Exercises: Literature Review [commonly 3–5 paragraphs]

- Begin by reading the example papers at the end of the chapter to gain a clearer understanding of how to write literature reviews for instrument development and testing studies.
- The literature review should synthesize the current published information regarding your instrument or a specific measurable construct so that readers can gain an understanding of what research has been completed to date.
- Then go to the literature and complete a database search about the instrument being assessed or, for a newly developed instrument, the instruments commonly used to measure a specific construct regarding functional performance. Identify all studies within a specified time period that directly relate to your topic.
- Synthesize the literature that you found for your readers. A synthesis means that you will summarize the existing literature using larger categories such as instrument, research design, specific population, sample size, findings, and limitations. It may be helpful for you to make a chart to organize this data so that you can present it in narrative form, highlighting commonalities and differences between studies.
- When only a handful (≤5) of studies exist, authors may present more specific information about each of these studies instead of synthesizing them as a group.
- Literature reviews should end with a paragraph about what information is missing from the existing literature and how your study intends to fill this gap in the profession's knowledge base.
- Ask a peer who understands research methods and who is familiar with your topic to read your literature review and provide feedback about its exhaustiveness and clarity.
- Make revisions based on the provided feedback.

Writing Exercises: Description of the Instrument [approximately 1–2 paragraphs]

- When an instrument has been newly developed, authors should state that the instrument was developed to meet an assessment need that was lacking for a specific clinical population.
- Authors should provide a description of the instrument that includes its purpose, intended population, and type of data collected (e.g., self-report, performance-based observer rating, Likert scale, open-ended questions, or total score yielding ratio data). If the instrument exists as another version(s), provide the psychometric properties of the other version(s).
- A more detailed description of the instrument will be provided in the Method section (including details such as administration length, number of instrument sections, number of items in each section, needed supplies and equipment, intended settings in which to administer the instrument, scoring procedures, and score range interpretations).
- A description of the theoretical bases used to develop the instrument should also be provided if the instrument is newly developed.

Final Paragraph Before Method [no heading]

The purpose statement is positioned in the final paragraph of the Introduction section. Here authors should clearly and concisely detail the need to establish specific psychometric properties of an instrument to help researchers and practitioners understand how well the assessment can be used to evaluate patient or participant performance. Either precise research questions or hypotheses should be provided. Research questions should include the targeted population, the instrument name (or names if convergent or criterion validity is examined), and the psychometric property or properties examined. Hypotheses should be formulated a priori (before data collection) and include the direction and magnitude of expectations.

The following are examples of good research questions for instrument development and testing studies:

- Is the Sensory Profile reliable for use with children with mental health diagnoses?
- What is the construct and content validity of the Evaluation of Social Skills Scale for Children with Autism?
- What is the convergent validity of two PTSD scales for veterans: Impact of Events Scale and Mississippi Scale for Combat-Related PTSD?

Writing Exercises: Purpose Statement

- See the example papers at the end of this chapter for a clearer understanding of how to write a purpose statement for an instrument development and testing study.

- Then practice writing a purpose statement for your manuscript.
- Begin with "The purpose of this study was to ..." and complete the sentence with the primary objective of your study.
- Example: "The purpose of the present study was to establish the content validity of the Visual Activity Card Sort for adolescents with autism spectrum disorder."
- Remember that all research reports are written in the past tense. Research proposals are written in future tense.

Writing Exercises: Research Questions

- See the example papers at the end of this chapter for a clearer understanding of how to write research questions for an instrument development and testing study.
- Practice writing research questions for your study using the provided guidelines.
- Make sure to include the targeted population, the instrument name (or names if convergent or criterion validity is examined), and the psychometric property or properties examined.
- Ask a peer to read your research questions and then explain what you are seeking through your study. If the reader is accurate, you have likely written good research questions. If they are not accurate, you may need to revise your research questions based on the labeling strategies outlined above.

Definitions

All new and unfamiliar terms that are presented in the Introduction (and throughout the text) should be defined when the term first appears in the manuscript. Common mistakes include failing to define terms, unclearly defining terms, presenting terms in one section and defining them in another, and changing the definition of a term in a paper. To understand how to write good definitions, authors should refer to Chapter 4.

Quotations

Quotations should only be used in scholarly writing when quoting a historical source or legal document; presenting a specific definition accepted by the scientific community, whose meaning would change if the exact wording were altered; and verbatim responses from patients or clients. With the exception of these instances, quotations should be avoided in health care writing. Authors should instead paraphrase and cite the original source.

A concise and well-written Introduction section should be approximately three to four double-spaced, typed pages in length.

Method

Research Design

Authors should begin the Method section with the subheading *Research Design*. Here, the specific design should be stated and described beyond simply noting that the study involved the assessment of psychometric properties. The specific types of reliability and/or validity assessed should be stated and defined, and authors should indicate whether the design is based on CTT or IRT. Authors must also indicate whether the design involves retrospective (i.e., data that have been collected as part of practice before the commencement of the study) or prospective (i.e., data that are collected as part of the present study) data collection. The Research Design section should end with a statement that the research study received institutional review board or ethics committee approval (or exemption) and that participants provided consent (for a prospective study).

Writing Exercises: Research Design [approximately 1 paragraph]

- See the example papers listed at the end of this chapter for a clearer understanding of how to write the Research Design subsection for an instrument development/testing study.
- Use the checklist at the end of this chapter to make an outline of your Research Design section.
- Write the Research Design section of your Methods, making sure to
  - Indicate the specific type of research design used (beyond stating that the study was a psychometric study).
  - State and define the specific types of reliability and/or validity that were assessed.
  - Indicate whether the design was based on CTT or IRT.
  - Indicate whether retrospective or prospective data were collected.
  - Indicate whether institutional review board or ethics committee approval was obtained or exempted.
  - Indicate whether participants provided consent.
- Ask a peer who understands research methods to read your Research Design section and let you know if it is clear and contains all needed information. Make revisions as needed.

Participants

The Participants subsection in the Method section details how and from where the participants were selected, the type of sampling method used, and inclusion and exclusion criteria. The Participants section allows readers to understand the characteristics of the targeted population rather than the actual sample that was enrolled and completed the study. In an instrument study, researchers must select a sample that adequately reflects the target population; otherwise, findings about instrument reliability and validity derived from a sample that does not match the intended population will be meaningless. For example, if researchers design an instrument for adults with mental health concerns but attempt to establish instrument reliability with healthy college students, reliability data derived from the sample of healthy college students will not yield genuine information about the instrument's reliability with adults with mental illness. The inclusion and exclusion criteria should be explicitly stated and, in a retrospective study, should detail how patient medical records were selected. Sampling methods and the settings from which participants were selected should be documented; such information is important for editors, reviewers, and readers to assess potential sampling bias and incongruence between the larger population and sample.

Writing Exercises: Participants [approximately 1–2 paragraphs]

- See the example papers listed at the end of this chapter to gain a clearer understanding of how to write the Participants subsection.
- Use the checklist at the end of this chapter to make an outline of your Participants section.
- Write the Participants section of your Methods, making sure to
  - Describe how participants were recruited and the sampling methods that were used to select them.
  - State who completed recruitment and describe the setting(s) from which participants were recruited.
  - Provide the precise inclusion/exclusion criteria for participant selection.
- Ask a peer who understands research methods to read your Participants section and describe who your targeted sample was, what sampling method was used to recruit your sample, from what setting(s) participants were recruited, and what the inclusion/exclusion criteria were.
- If your reader could easily identify these, you have likely written a strong Participants section. If they could not, revise your Participants section using the above guidelines. Repeat the process of obtaining feedback and making revisions.

Instruments

Although the instrument assessed in the study was introduced in the Introduction, authors must provide specific details about it in this section. The following should have been documented in the Introduction: the instrument purpose, intended population, and type of data collected (e.g., self-report, performance-based observer rating, Likert scale, open-ended questions, or total score yielding ratio data). In the Methods section, document details such as the instrument's administration length, number of instrument sections and subsections, number of items in each section, needed supplies and equipment, intended settings in which the instrument was meant to be administered, scoring procedures, score range interpretations, whether and what type of training is needed to administer the instrument, and what professionals possess the skills needed for instrument administration. The setting in which the instrument was intended to be administered should be described, particularly because performance-based instruments should be used in real-life activities within the community to obtain genuine information about patient daily function. If any previous psychometric properties regarding reliability, validity, and responsiveness were established, these should be noted with citations. When convergent and criterion validity are assessed, the comparison instrument should be described in detail with regard to the above information.

Writing Exercises: Instruments [approximately 1–3 paragraphs]

- See the example papers listed at the end of this chapter to gain a clearer understanding of how to write the Instruments subsection for an instrument development/testing study.
- Then use the checklist at the end of this chapter to make an outline of your Instruments section.
- Using your outline, write the Instruments section of your Methods, making sure to
  - Describe the instrument with regard to the instrument's administration length, number of instrument sections and subsections, number of items in each section, needed supplies and equipment, intended settings in which the instrument was meant to be administered, scoring procedures, score range interpretations, whether and what type of training is needed to administer the instrument, and what professionals possess the skills needed for instrument administration.
  - Provide information about previously established psychometric properties regarding reliability, validity, and responsiveness. List numeric values, statistical test values, exact *p* values, and confidence intervals where appropriate. Provide citations for all psychometric studies.
  - When convergent and criterion validity are assessed, the comparison instrument should be described in detail with regard to the above information.
- Ask a peer who understands instrument development and testing to read your Instruments section and let you know if they can describe the instrument's unique characteristics and properties noted in the first indented bullet above. If the reader cannot, ask what is unclear and use that feedback to revise your work. Repeat the process of obtaining feedback and making revisions.

Procedures

The Procedures subsection should document the process of instrument development, revision, or translation (if applicable); the procedures through which reliability, validity, and/or responsiveness were assessed; the study timeline and sequence of events; and the setting in which instrument administration occurred.

Content Validity

In a content validity study, authors should indicate whether an assessment was performed to determine the following:

- Whether all test items refer to relevant aspects of the construct and collectively reflect the construct

- Whether all items are relevant for the study population with regard to age, gender, disease characteristics, geographical region/country, and setting
- Whether a table of specifications was used to determine the number, range, and content of instrument items
- Whether a panel of content experts was used to assess content validity

Convergent and Criterion Validity

- In a convergent or criterion validity study, authors should document the steps used to ensure that the comparison instrument was a reasonable gold standard or best available instrument for comparison.
- In such studies, evaluators should be anonymized to the other measures to minimize the risk of expectation and limit biased ratings.

Reliability

For assessment of reliability, including interrater, intrarater, and test–retest, authors should report the following:

- Whether at least two measurements were available for comparison
- Whether the instrument administrations were independent of each other—the first administration did not influence the second
- The time interval between instrument administrations (2 weeks is customary for most reliability studies and is considered long enough to reduce the risk of item recall but short enough to limit the possibility that the patient did not maintain stability on the construct being measured)
- Whether patients were stable on the construct measured over the 2-week period of instrument administration
- Whether conditions were the same for both instrument administrations (i.e., setting, type of instructions provided)
- For interrater reliability, whether raters were anonymized to each other's scores to reduce bias

For internal consistency—the degree to which all instrument items reflect the same underlying construct—authors should report whether scale unidimensionality was checked. Scale unidimensionality refers to the degree to which a scale measures one construct.

Translation Studies

When an instrument has been translated into another language, authors should indicate the following:

- The expertise level of the translators with regard to language translation, knowledge of the diagnosis, and knowledge of the construct measured by the instrument
- Whether the translators worked independently of each other
- Whether back and forward translations were performed
- How differences between the original and translated instrument versions were resolved

- Whether the translation was reviewed by a panel of experts
- Whether the translated instrument was pretested to check for possible problems in interpretation, cultural relevance, and understandability

Writing Exercises: Procedures [approximately 3–4 paragraphs]

- See the example papers listed at the end of this chapter to gain a clearer understanding of how to write the Procedures subsection for an instrument development/testing study.
- Then use the checklist at the end of this chapter to make an outline of your Procedures section.
- Using your outline, write the Procedures section of your Methods, making sure to
  - Report the steps of the study in sufficient detail so that it can be evaluated and replicated by readers.
  - Indicate who was responsible for and implemented each procedural step.
  - Document the process of instrument development, revision, or translation.
  - Document the procedures through which reliability, validity, and/or responsiveness were assessed.
  - Detail the study timeline and sequence of events.
  - Describe the setting in which instrument administration occurred.
- Ask a peer who understands instrument development to read your procedures section and describe it back to you, indicating what is clear and what needs greater clarification. Make revisions based on this feedback. Repeat the process of obtaining feedback and making revisions.

Data Collection

In the Data Collection subsection, authors should describe the sequence of the data collection schedule and how and by whom data were collected. Data collectors should be described in terms of type of professional, expertise level, and training in data collection procedures. Such elements are critical for editors, reviewers, and readers to evaluate whether data collection may have been biased by differences among data collector training and experience. Anonymization is a crucial element used to reduce the risk that data collectors were influenced by each other, separate test administrations, and participant scores.

- In convergent and criterion validity studies, authors should indicate whether data collectors were anonymized to the other instrument and participant scores to reduce expectation bias.
- In interrater reliability studies, authors should indicate whether data collectors were anonymized to each other's scores.

Writing Exercises: Data Collection [approximately 2–3 paragraphs]

- See the example papers at the end of this chapter for a clearer understanding of how to write the Data Collection subsection of an instrument development/ testing study.
- Then use the checklist at the end of this chapter to make an outline of the main points in your Data Collection section.
- Write the Data Collection section of your Methods, making sure to
  - Report the data collection schedule with regard to the sequence of data collection and how and by whom data were collected.
  - Describe data collectors with regard to type of professional, expertise level, and training in data collection procedures.
  - In convergent and criterion validity studies, indicate whether data collectors were anonymized to the other instrument and participant scores to reduce expectation bias.
  - In interrater reliability studies, indicate whether data collectors were anonymized to each other's scores.
- Ask a peer who understands research methods to read your Data Collection section and describe it back to you, indicating what is clear and what needs greater clarification. Make revisions based on that feedback. Repeat the process of obtaining feedback and making revisions.

Data Analysis

In instrument development and testing studies, authors must indicate whether data analysis was based on CTT or IRT, as this will determine the appropriateness of the selected statistical models and tests. When using CTT, authors should describe and cite all statistical test methods. The use of nontraditional statistical procedures that are incongruent with traditional parametric and nonparametric data analysis should be justified and cited. The use of statistical tests that may be congruent with traditional parametric and nonparametric data analysis but are likely unfamiliar to readers should also be justified and cited. Authors should identify and cite the software program used to generate statistical analysis and indicate at what significance level probability was set.

When using IRT, authors should describe the model (e.g., one-parameter logistic model, OPLM; partial credit model, PCM; graded response model, GRM) and the software program (e.g., RUMM2020, WINSTEPS, OPLM, MULTILOG, PARSCALE, BILOG, NLMIXED). Authors should also report the method of estimation used (e.g., conditional maximum likelihood (CML); marginal maximum likelihood (MML)) and identify the assumptions for estimating parameters of the IRT model (unidimensionality; local independence; item fit; and differential item functioning (DIF)).

Writing Exercises: Data Analysis [approximately 2–3 paragraphs]

- See the example papers at the end of this chapter for a clearer understanding of how to write the Data Analysis subsection.
- Then use the checklist at the end of this chapter to make an outline of the main points in your Data Analysis section.
- Write the Data Analysis section of your Methods, making sure to
  - For CIT:
    - Describe and cite all statistical test methods.
    - Justify and cite the use of nontraditional statistical procedures that differ from traditional parametric and nonparametric data analysis procedures.
    - Justify and cite the use of statistical tests that may be congruent with traditional parametric and nonparametric data analysis but are likely unfamiliar to readers.
    - Identify and cite the software program used for statistical analysis.
    - Indicate at what significance level probability was set.
  - For IRT:
    - Describe the IRT model used.
    - Name and cite the software program used.
    - Report the method of estimation used.
    - Identify the assumptions for estimating parameters of the IRT model.
- Ask a peer who understands instrument development/testing to read your Data Analysis section and describe it back to you, indicating what is clear and what needs greater clarification. Make revisions based on that feedback. Repeat the process of obtaining feedback and making revisions.

A concise and well-written Method section should be approximately four to five double-spaced, typed pages in length.

Results

Although most instrument development and testing studies in education and social science do not report information about participant flow, information about the number of participants who withdrew (or were withdrawn by the researcher) because they could not tolerate test conditions is critical in the reporting of health care instruments. The Results section should begin with information about participant flow (particularly the number enrolled, the number withdrawn due to intolerance of testing conditions and why, and the final sample size) and participant demographics. Participant demographics should be reported in terms of age, gender, race, ethnicity, education level, socioeconomic level, and topic-specific characteristics such as functional status. Demographics should be reported in absolute numbers; if percentages are provided, the absolute number from which the percentage was derived should also be reported. The reporting of participant demographics is critical for readers to evaluate whether your sample matched the larger population; if it did not, psychometric properties reported in the study will be meaningless. After the reporting of final sample size, authors can describe power analyses, sample size estimations, and confidence level estimations that were calculated to ensure that the study sample size was adequate to yield reliable statistical results. It is important to acknowledge the number of missing items and describe the protocol for handling missing items (*missing items* refers to either the average number of missing items per instrument or the percentage of missing responses per item).

The remainder of the Results section consists of a reporting of your findings and should be organized in accordance with the order of research questions or hypotheses outlined in the purpose section of the Introduction. Findings should be reported for each research question without interpretation. Results should be reported using statistical test values, p values, and confidence intervals.

See Chapter 10, Reporting Statistical Data in Text and Tables, to understand how to correctly report statistical tests and symbols in the Results section.

Writing Exercises: Results [approximately 1–3 double-spaced, typed pages]

- See the example papers at the end of this chapter for a clearer understanding of how to write the Results section for an instrument development/testing study.
- Then use the checklist at the end of this chapter to make an outline of the main points in your Results section.
- In your outline, first include information about participant flow and demographics.
- Then order your research questions in accordance with the order listed in the Introduction. Beneath each question, insert the primary points that you want to include.
- Using your outline, write the Results section, making sure to
  - Begin the Results section with information about participant flow and demographics. Provide the final sample size. Report information about the number of participants who withdrew because they could not tolerate test conditions (and why).
  - Report all findings without interpreting them.
  - Report results in absolute numbers rather than percentages. When percentages are provided, indicate the absolute numbers from which the percentages were derived.
  - Report power analyses, sample size estimations, and confidence level estimations that were calculated to ensure that the sample size was adequate to yield reliable results.
  - Acknowledge the number of missing items and describe the protocol for handling missing items.
  - Report results using statistical test values, p values, and confidence intervals.
- Finally, ask a peer who understands instrument design to read your Results section and describe it back to you, indicating what is clear and what needs greater clarification. Make revisions based on that feedback. Repeat the process of obtaining feedback and making revisions until the Results section has all needed information and is clear.

A concisely and well-written Results section should be approximately one to three double-spaced, typed pages in length, depending on the number of psychometric properties addressed in the study.

Discussion

The Discussion section provides the opportunity for authors to interpret findings about the instrument's psychometric properties. It is important that authors not overstate their findings but rather report results with caution and acknowledge study limitations such as sample size insufficiency. Authors should refrain from using exemplars or qualifiers (such as *excellent*) when interpreting the psychometric properties of the assessed instrument. It is more appropriate to use the terms *low*, *moderate*, and *high* and allow readers to independently interpret the numeric values of statistical tests. The Discussion section should be organized in accordance with the research questions or hypotheses stated in the Introduction and Results sections. Authors should answer each research question or hypothesis based on study findings and report whether findings are novel, support previous studies, or challenge previously established information about an instrument's properties and use.

Writing Exercises: Discussion [approximately 3–4 double-spaced, typed pages]

- See the example papers listed at the end of this chapter for a clearer understanding of how to write the Discussion section.
- Then use the checklist at the end of this chapter to make an outline of the main points in your Discussion section.
- Begin by ordering your research questions in accordance with the order of research questions addressed in your Results section. Beneath each question, insert the primary points of the Discussion that you want to include.
- Make sure to
    - Explain and interpret all findings without repeating the results. Why might each finding have occurred? Be cautious not to overstate findings.
    - Indicate whether findings are novel, support previous studies, or challenge previously established information about an instrument's properties and use.
- Use your outline to write a first draft of your Discussion section.
- Once drafted, ask a peer who understands instrument design to read your Discussion section and describe it back to you, indicating what is clear and what needs greater clarification. Make revisions based on that feedback. Repeat the process of obtaining feedback and making revisions.

Limitations

In the Limitations subsection, authors should acknowledge the weaknesses of the study that may have biased results. Common limitations in an instrument development/testing study include small sample size (that was insufficient for statistical power), use of convenience samples, missing data, compromised anonymization procedures, failure to use a panel of experts in content validity studies, and failure to determine that patients remained stable on the construct being measured in the interval between measurements (in reliability studies). Authors should discuss the generalizability of the sample to the larger population and address differences between the target population and the study sample.

Writing Exercises: Limitations [approximately 1–2 paragraphs]

- See the example papers listed at the end of this chapter for a clearer understanding of how to write the Limitations subsection of an instrument development/testing study.
- Then use the checklist at the end of this chapter to make an outline of the main points in your Limitations section.
- Write a first draft of the Limitations section, making sure to
  - Acknowledge all possible limitations that may have biased study results (e.g., small sample size, use of convenience samples, missing data, compromised anonymization procedures, failure to use genuine experts on a panel of experts in content validity studies, and failure to determine that patients remained stable on the construct being measured in the interval between measurements in reliability studies).
  - Describe differences between the target population and the study sample; discuss how these may have impacted the generalizability of findings.
- Ask a peer who understands instrument development/testing to read your Limitations section and describe it back to you, indicating what is clear and what needs greater clarification. Make revisions based on that feedback. Repeat the process of obtaining feedback and making revisions.

Future Research

In the Future Research subsection, authors should suggest ways in which the above limitations can be addressed in more rigorous studies and identify research questions that remain unanswered concerning the instrument's development, refinement, and use with the intended population.

Writing Exercises: Future Research [approximately 1–2 paragraphs]

- See the example papers listed at the end of this chapter for a clearer understanding of how to write the Future Research subsection of instrument development/testing studies.
- Then use the checklist at the end of this chapter to make an outline of the main points in your Future Research section.

- Write a first draft of the Future Research section, making sure to
  - Describe how future research can address the study's limitations.
  - Identify research questions that remain unanswered concerning the instrument's development, refinement, and use with the intended population, and suggest directions for future studies.
- Ask a peer who understands instrument development/testing to read your Future Research section and describe it back to you, indicating what is clear and what needs greater clarification. Make revisions based on that feedback. Repeat the process of obtaining feedback and making revisions.

Implications for Practice

In this manuscript section, authors should recommend how the instrument should be used in practice with regard to its present developmental stage. Practitioners and researchers will best benefit from a brief discussion about the instrument's reliable and valid use with specific populations and settings. A concise, well-written Implications for Practice section should be approximately 4–6 bullets or 250–300 words.

Writing Exercises: Implications for Practice [approximately 6 bullets or 1 paragraph]

- See the example papers listed at the end of this chapter for a clearer understanding of how to write the Implications for Practice subsection of the Discussion.
- Then use the checklist at the end of this chapter to make an outline of the main points in your Implications for Practice section.
- Write a first draft of the Implications for Practice section, making sure to cautiously suggest how study findings may be used to inform clinical practice.
- Ask a peer who understands instrument development/testing to read your Implications for Practice section and describe it back to you, indicating what is clear and what needs greater clarification. Ask the reader to comment on whether you may have overstated your findings' application to practice. Make revisions based on that feedback. Repeat the process of obtaining feedback and making revisions.

Conclusion

In this final manuscript section, authors should summarize findings about the instrument's properties and recommended use based on the present study's findings, identify questions about the instrument that have yet to be answered regarding psychometric properties and clinical use, and recommend next steps in the instrument's development. A concise, well-written Conclusion section should be approximately 250–300 words.

Writing Exercises: Conclusion [approximately 1–2 paragraphs]

- See the example papers listed at the end of this chapter for a clearer understanding of how to write the Conclusion subsection.
- Then use the checklist at the end of this chapter to make an outline of the main points in your Conclusion section.
- Write a first draft of the Conclusion section, making sure to
  - Summarize the study's primary findings about the instrument's properties and recommended use, identify questions about the instrument that have yet to be answered regarding psychometric properties and clinical use, and recommend next steps in the instrument's development.
  - Make sure not to overstate study findings.
- Ask a peer who understands research manuscript writing to read your Conclusion section and describe it back to you, indicating what is clear and what needs greater clarification.
- Ask the reader to comment on whether you may have overstated your findings or their application to practice. Make revisions based on that feedback. Repeat the process of obtaining feedback and making revisions.

A concisely and well-written Discussion section should be approximately four to five double-spaced, typed pages in length in its entirety (all subsections combined).

After the end of the Conclusion section, the following are the remaining manuscript sections in the order in which they should be presented in the paper:

- References
- Tables
- Figures

Checklist for Manuscript Structure and Content of Instrument Development and Testing Studies

Title

☐ Include the following: population, instrument name, or construct measured, and psychometric properties assessed.

Abstract

☐ Objectives: In one to two sentences, describe the purpose of the study, which will address the development or further refinement of an instrument and/or the assessment of its psychometric properties.

☐ Method: In one to two sentences, provide information about the research design, study timeline, participants (population, sample size), and data collection procedures.

☐ Results: In one to two sentences, report the primary findings along with statistical test results as calculated using either CTT or IRT.

- ☐ Conclusions: In one to two sentences, describe the implications of findings for the instrument's use with the targeted population.

Introduction

- ☐ Describe the background of the problem as it relates to the population, profession, and society.
- ☐ Report the incidence of the targeted population.
- ☐ Describe the impact of the diagnosis or clinical problem on functional community participation.
- ☐ Define the construct measured by the instrument.
- ☐ Define all novel or unfamiliar terms directly when first mentioned.
- ☐ Describe the need for the instrument.
- ☐ Literature Review: Discuss the literature examining how the construct has been measured in the targeted population using other instruments.
- ☐ Provide a brief description of the instrument (a detailed description will be made in the Method section). Include the instrument's purpose, intended population, and type of data collected (e.g., self-report, performance-based observer rating, Likert scale, open-ended questions, or total score yielding ratio data).
- ☐ Describe the theoretical base for an instrument that is newly developed.
- ☐ Purpose statement: detail the need to establish specific psychometric properties for the instrument.
- ☐ Provide precise research questions or a priori hypotheses (include the direction and magnitude of expectations for all hypotheses).

Method

Research Design

- ☐ Indicate the specific type of research design used (beyond stating that the study is a psychometric study).
- ☐ State and define the specific types of reliability and/or validity that were assessed.
- ☐ Indicate whether the design is based on CTT or IRT.
- ☐ Indicate whether retrospective or prospective data have been collected.
- ☐ Indicate whether institutional review board or ethics committee approval was obtained or exempted.
- ☐ Indicate whether participants provided consent.

Participants

- ☐ Describe the sampling method and setting(s) from which participants were selected.
- ☐ Describe the inclusion and exclusion criteria so that readers can understand the characteristics of the target population.

Instruments

- ☐ Describe the instrument with regard to the instrument's administration length, number of instrument sections and subsections, number of items in each section, needed supplies and equipment, intended settings in which the instrument was meant to be administered, scoring procedures, score range interpretations, whether and what type of training is needed to administer the instrument, and which professionals possess the skills needed for instrument administration.

- ☐ Provide information about previously established psychometric properties regarding reliability, validity, and responsiveness (provide citations for all psychometric studies).
- ☐ When convergent and criterion validity are assessed, the comparison instrument should be described in detail with regard to the above information.

Procedures

- ☐ Document the process of instrument development, revision, or translation.
- ☐ Document the procedures through which reliability, validity, and/or responsiveness were assessed.
- ☐ Detail the study timeline and sequence of events.
- ☐ Describe the setting in which instrument administration occurred.

For Content Validity Studies

- ☐ Indicate whether an assessment was performed to determine the following:
  - ☐ Whether all test items refer to relevant aspects of the construct and collectively reflect the construct
  - ☐ Whether all items are relevant for the study population with regard to age, gender, disease characteristics, geographical region or country, and setting
  - ☐ Whether a table of specifications was used to determine the number, range, and content of instrument items
  - ☐ Whether a panel of content experts was used to assess content validity

For Convergent and Criterion Validity Studies

- ☐ Document the steps used to ensure that the comparison instrument was a reasonable gold standard or best available instrument for comparison.
- ☐ Indicate whether evaluators were anonymized to the other measures to minimize the risk of expectation and limit biased ratings.

For Reliability Studies

- ☐ For assessment of reliability, including interrater, intrarater, and test–retest, report the following:
  - ☐ Whether at least two measurements were available for comparison
  - ☐ Whether the instrument administrations were independent of each other—the first administration did not influence the second
  - ☐ The time interval between instrument administrations (2 weeks is customary for most reliability studies and is considered long enough to reduce the risk of item recall but short enough to limit the possibility that the patient did not maintain stability on the construct being measured)
  - ☐ Whether patients were stable on the construct measured over the 2-week period of instrument administration
  - ☐ Whether conditions were the same for both instrument administrations (i.e., setting, type of instructions provided)

  - ☐ For interrater reliability, whether raters were anonymized to each other's scores to reduce bias
- ☐ For internal consistency, report whether scale unidimensionality was checked.

For Translation Studies

- ☐ When an instrument has been translated into another language, indicate the following:
  - ☐ The expertise level of the translators with regard to language translation, knowledge of the diagnosis, and knowledge of the construct measured by the instrument
  - ☐ Whether the translators worked independently of each other
  - ☐ Whether back and forward translation were performed
  - ☐ How differences between the original and translated instrument versions were resolved
  - ☐ Whether the translation was reviewed by a panel of experts
  - ☐ Whether the translated instrument was pretested to check for possible problems in interpretation, cultural relevance, and understandability

Data Collection

- ☐ Report the data collection schedule with regard to the sequence of data collection and how and by whom data were collected.
- ☐ Describe data collectors with regard to type of professional, expertise level, and training in data collection procedures.
- ☐ In convergent and criterion validity studies, indicate whether data collectors were anonymized to the other instrument and participant scores to reduce expectation bias.
- ☐ In interrater reliability studies, indicate whether data collectors were anonymized to each other's scores.

Data Analysis

- ☐ Report whether data analysis was based on CTT or IRT.
- ☐ For CTT:
  - ☐ Describe and cite all statistical test methods.
  - ☐ Justify and cite the use of nontraditional statistical procedures that are incongruent with traditional parametric and nonparametric data analysis.
  - ☐ Justify and cite the use of statistical tests that may be congruent with traditional parametric and nonparametric data analysis but are likely unfamiliar to readers.
  - ☐ Identify and cite the software program used to generate statistical analysis.
  - ☐ Indicate at what significance level probability was set.
- ☐ For IRT:
  - ☐ Describe the IRT model used (e.g., one-parameter logistic model, OPLM; partial credit model, PCM; graded response model, GRM).
  - ☐ Name and cite the software program used (e.g., RUMM2020, WINSTEPS, OPLM, MULTILOG, PARSCALE, BILOG, NLMIXED).

- ☐ Report the method of estimation used (e.g., CML and MML).
- ☐ Identify the assumptions for estimating parameters of the IRT model (unidimensionality; local independence; item fit; and DIF).

Results

- ☐ Provide the final sample size.
- ☐ Report information about the number of participants who withdrew because they could not tolerate test conditions (and why).
- ☐ Report participant demographics with regard to age, gender, race, ethnicity, education level, socioeconomic level, and topic-specific characteristics such as functional status.
- ☐ Describe power analyses, sample size estimations, and confidence level estimations that were calculated to ensure that the study sample size was adequate to yield reliable statistical results.
- ☐ Acknowledge the number of missing items and describe the protocol for handling missing items.
- ☐ Organize and report findings in accordance with the order of research questions or hypotheses outlined in the Introduction section.
- ☐ Report results using statistical test values, *p* values, and confidence intervals.

Discussion

- ☐ Organize and provide interpretations of findings in accordance with the order of research questions or hypotheses outlined in the Results section.
- ☐ Be cautious not to overstate findings.
- ☐ Indicate whether findings are novel, support previous studies, or challenge previously established information about an instrument's properties and use.

Limitations

- ☐ Acknowledge limitations such as small sample size, use of convenience samples, missing data, compromised anonymization procedures, failure to use actual experts on a panel of experts in content validity studies, and failure to determine that patients remained stable on the construct being measured in the interval between measurements (in reliability studies).
- ☐ Discuss the generalizability of the sample to the larger population and address differences between the target population and the study sample.

Future Research

- ☐ Suggest ways in which limitations can be addressed in more rigorous studies.
- ☐ Identify research questions that remain unanswered concerning the instrument's development, refinement, and use with the intended population.

Implications for Practice

- ☐ Recommend how the instrument should be used in practice with regard to its present developmental stage.

Conclusion

- ☐ Summarize the study's primary findings about the instrument's properties and recommended use.
- ☐ Identify questions about the instrument that have yet to be answered regarding psychometric properties and clinical use.
- ☐ Recommend next steps in the instrument's development.

Examples of Well-Written Instrument Development and Testing Studies

Gutman, S., O'Day, K., Choi, A., Kearney, A., & Rogers, S. (2023). Establishing initial content validity, interrater reliability, and intra-rater reliability of the revised visual activity sort for at-risk adolescents and young adults. *Open Journal of Occupational Therapy, 11*(4), 1–15. https://doi.org/10.15453/2168-6408.2156

Rosenblum, S., Josman, N., & Toglia, J. (2017). Development of the Daily Living Questionnaire (DLQ): A factor analysis study. *Open Journal of Occupational Therapy, 5*(4). https://doi.org/10.15453/2168-6408.1326

References

American Psychological Association. (2020). *Publication manual of the American Psychological Association* (7th ed.). Author.

Gagnier, J. J., de Arruda, G. T., Terwee, C. B., & Mokkink, L. B. (2025). COSMIN reporting guideline for studies on measurement properties of patient-reported outcome measures: Version 2.0. *Quality of Life Research*, *34*, 1901–1911. https://doi.org/10.1007/s11136-025-03950-x

CHAPTER 7

Manuscript Structure and Content for Needs Assessments

A needs assessment is a systematic gathering of information necessary to understand the clinical needs of an emerging population for which occupational therapy services have not been traditionally provided. Examples of emerging populations that could benefit from occupational therapy services, but who have not typically received such services, include (a) young adults with intellectual disabilities who have reached an age when mandated services end but who are struggling to transition to the adult roles of worker, post-secondary student, and independent community dweller; (b) homeless adults (and their children) who require daily life skills needed to transition from the shelter to supported or independent housing; and (c) adolescents in low socioeconomic school systems who are at-risk for school failure and would benefit from assistance to succeed academically, learn needed daily life skills, and plan for the transition to post-secondary education/employment. The surveying of a population's needs is often implemented through interviews, questionnaires, and focus groups.

Needs assessments commonly make good capstone projects because they provide important information for the profession and are able to be completed in a shorter period of time than traditional research studies. If a needs assessment is completed as a capstone project, it does not need institutional review board approval unless authors wish to publish the data. The reporting of a needs assessment is achieved through a type of manuscript design in which the procedures and findings are documented methodically in an APA-style (2020) paper with specific headings. These headings are provided below.

Manuscript Headings and Formatting for Needs Assessments

Title

Begin the paper with a title on a separate title page. The title should be centered, bolded, and typed in uppercase and lowercase letters.

DOI: 10.4324/9781003734550-7

Abstract

The Abstract should be placed on the page directly following the title page. The word *Abstract* should be capitalized, centered, and bolded. The *A* in Abstract should be capitalized. If keywords are required, they are inserted directly after the abstract and indented. The term *keywords* is italicized, capitalized, and indented:

Keywords: stroke, community participation, activities of daily living

Introduction

The Introduction begins on the page directly following the Abstract. The heading *Introduction* is not typed in the manuscript because the beginning of the manuscript text alerts the reader that the Introduction has begun.

Literature Review

In capstone projects, the Literature Review is commonly a new section that follows the Introduction and is labeled with a separate heading that is capitalized, bolded, and flush left. If the capstone project is being turned into a format for publication, the Literature Review may be shortened and embedded within the Introduction without a separate heading.

Method

The Method section is positioned directly after the Introduction. The heading *Method* is centered, capitalized, and bolded.

Needs Assessment Design

Needs Assessment Design is the first subheading in the Method section. It is capitalized, bolded, and flush left.

Participant Selection

Participant Selection is the second subheading in the Method section. It is capitalized, bolded, and flush left.

Instruments

Instruments is the third subheading in the Method section. It is capitalized, bolded, and flush left.

Procedures

Procedures is the fourth subheading in the Method sections. It is capitalized, bolded, and flush left.

Data Collection

Data Collection is the subheading that directly follows Procedures. It is capitalized, bolded, and flush left.

Data Analysis

Data Analysis is the subheading that directly follows Data Collection. It is capitalized, bolded, and flush left.

Results

The Results section directly follows the Data Analysis subheading and begins a new section of the paper. The heading *Results* is capitalized, bolded, and centered.

Discussion

The Discussion section directly follows the Results and begins a new section of the paper. The heading *Discussion* is capitalized, bolded, and centered.

Limitations

The Limitations section is a subsection of the Discussion and has its own subheading. The subheading *Limitations* is capitalized, bolded, and flush left.

Future Directions [or Future Research]

The Future Directions subsection directly follows the Limitations subsection. The heading *Future Directions* is used when the needs assessment is not carried out as a research study. When the needs assessment is completed as a research study, the heading *Future Research* should be used. The subheading *Future Directions* (or *Future Research*) is bolded, capitalized, and flush left.

Implications for Practice

The Implications for Practice section is a subsection of the Discussion and follows the Future Directions section. The heading is capitalized, bolded, and flush left.

Conclusion

The Conclusion is the final subsection of the Discussion and follows Implications for Practice. The heading is capitalized, bolded, and flush left.

References

References begin on a separate page following the Conclusion. The heading is centered, capitalized, and bolded.

Tables

Tables should be provided after the end of the references and should begin on a separate page. Each table should be presented on its own page. Tables are named and presented in accordance with the order in which they are mentioned in the text. The title of the Table is inserted beneath the Table heading:

Table 1 [bolded, capitalized, and flush left]
Participant Demographics [italicized, capitalized, and flush left]

Figures

Figures should be provided after the end of the Tables and begin on a separate page. Each figure should be presented on its own page. Figures are named and presented in accordance with the order in which they are mentioned in the text. The title of the Figure is inserted beneath the Figure heading:

Figure 1 [bolded, capitalized, and flush left]
Examples of Participant Quotes [italicized, capitalized, and flush left]

Manuscript Heading Content for Needs Assessments

A needs assessment manuscript should be approximately 5000 words in length, double-spaced.

There should be no repetition of content in the paper. The below sections and subsections should not contain overlap and, if written as suggested, will not.

Title

Titles help readers understand paper content. If published, titles help indexers categorize articles so that they can be easily accessed. If critical information is missing from titles, articles may never be accessed by their intended audience. The title of a needs assessment should concisely describe the topic and identify the main variables examined.

Needs assessment titles should contain two essential elements:

1. The population's diagnosis/condition and age or developmental level
2. An indication that the project was an examination of a population's needs; the words *needs assessment* (the design) should be inserted in the title

Examples of good needs assessment titles include the following:

- The Community Mobility Needs of Seniors Post-Stroke Who Have Stopped Driving: A Needs Assessment
- A Needs Assessment of Adults with ADHD Who are Striving to Juggle Work and Family Responsibilities
- A Needs Assessment of Women Who Became Homeless as a Result of Domestic Violence
- A Needs Assessment of Families Raising Nonverbal Children with Autism Spectrum Disorder

Abbreviations in the title should be avoided unless commonly used and understood in the health care community.

Writing Exercises: Titles

- Practice writing a title for your needs assessment using the above guidelines.
- Make sure to include
  - The population's diagnosis or condition
  - The population's age or developmental level
  - A statement that the project was an examination of a population's needs
  - The words *needs assessment* (the design) should be inserted in the title
- Ask a peer (who does not know about your project) to read your title and describe what they think your paper is about. If they are correct, you have likely written an adequate title. If they are not correct, you may need to revise your title using the above directions.
- If revision is needed, make changes and repeat the process of seeking feedback with another peer.

Abstract

Unless otherwise specified by a journal's author guidelines, needs assessments should summarize the manuscript content using the abstract subheadings (a) objectives, (b) method, (c) results, and (d) conclusions. Using these subheadings will ensure that you provide the reader with critical information needed to understand manuscript content and select papers from database searches. For a capstone project, abstracts should be no more than 200 words. If submitting to a journal, authors should check and adhere to the word count specifications outlined in the journal's author guidelines.

The following subheadings should be used in the abstract.

- Objectives: In 1–2 sentences, authors should describe the purpose of the needs assessment. In a needs assessment, the purpose will address the systematic collection of data regarding a population's clinical needs in order to design intervention and inform future practice decisions.
- Method: In 1–2 sentences, authors should provide information about the population (diagnosis/condition, age group, functional status), sample size, needs assessment design (e.g., one-to-one interview, online questionnaire, focus group), and the setting from which patients/clients were selected.
- Results: In 1–2 sentences, authors should summarize findings about the sample's needs gleaned from data collection (interview, questionnaire, focus group).
- Conclusions: In 1–2 sentences, authors should describe the implications of the needs assessment findings with regard to how these preliminary findings can be used to inform practice for their sample in the sample's own homes and communities.

Writing Exercises: Abstracts [approximately 200 words]

- See the example papers at the end of this chapter to gain a clearer understanding of how to write abstracts.

- The abstract is the last section that should be written after all other manuscript sections are completed.
- Practice writing an abstract for your needs assessment using the outlined guidelines.
- Objectives: Go to the purpose statement of your paper and identify the purpose of the project. Modify this sentences(s) so that it is not taken verbatim from the paper text.
- Method: Go to the Methods section of your paper and identify information regarding the following: participants (e.g., population, sample size, recruitment), needs assessment design, and data collection procedures. Revise these sentences so that they are not written verbatim and can be shortened and combined into one to two sentences.
- Results: Select the primary findings from your Results section. You will likely not be able to report all of your findings in the abstract. Select approximately two primary results that are most salient to your project. Try to rewrite these sentences so that they are shortened into one to two sentences. If statistical analysis was used, each result should be accompanied by the statistical test result, exact *p* value, and confidence interval.
- Conclusions: Go to your Discussion section and select one to two primary points regarding the implications of your findings for the sample and their clinical or community setting. Rewrite these sentences so that they are shortened into one to two sentences.
- Ask a peer to read your abstract and let you know if it is clear, and if not, what can be made clearer.
- If needed, write a second draft and repeat the process of obtaining feedback and making revisions.

Introduction

The Introduction begins on the page directly following the abstract. The heading *Introduction* is not typed in the paper because the beginning of the paper text alerts the reader that the Introduction has begun.

The Introduction of a needs assessment should be four to five double-spaced, typed pages.

The Introduction should provide background information about the population and the problems they may encounter with regard to clinical course, function in daily life, and community participation. Background information relating to incidence or prevalence should also be provided. The implication of the population's problems, as they may impact the larger society, should be discussed. The author should also indicate how the population's problems may be relevant to and *potentially* addressable by the profession.

The need for the project should be made clear and answer the question, "Why is this project needed now?" Usually, the need for the project relates to the importance of understanding the clinical needs of a population that traditionally does not receive occupational therapy services but that could potentially benefit from them.

Writing Exercises: Introduction [4–5 double-spaced pages]

- See the example papers at the end of this chapter to understand how to write clear Introduction sections.

Background [approximately 2–3 paragraphs]

- Practice writing the Introduction section of your needs assessment.
- Begin by describing the background of the problem as it relates to the clinical population addressed. Most backgrounds begin with information about the prevalence or incidence rate of the addressed clinical condition.
- Describe the current problem with regard to the clinical population's daily life function, community participation, or some other important aspect of their life situation. How have these factors impacted the addressed clinical population?
- Then describe how this problem has impacted the larger society and the profession.

Need for Project [commonly 2 paragraphs]

- The need for the project answers the questions, "Why is this project needed now to help the addressed clinical population?" "How will this study contribute to the knowledge needed to inform clinical practice to assist this population?" For a needs assessment, the need for the project often addresses the obtaining of knowledge about the potential clinical needs of an emerging population that has traditionally not received occupational therapy services but that could benefit from them.
- Ask a peer to read your Introduction and describe the background and need for your project. If they could not adequately describe the background and need as you intended, identify what they missed and rewrite those components.
- Write a second draft and repeat the process of obtaining feedback and making revisions.

Literature Review

In capstone projects, the Literature Review is a new section that follows the Introduction and is labeled with a separate heading. In a needs assessment, the literature review should focus on interventions that have been used by other professions to assist this population, the effectiveness of those interventions, and what is missing but needed by the population to attain optimal community participation. If no attempts to provide assistance to the population have been made by other professions, authors should clearly state this. Authors should make clear how occupational therapists could potentially contribute to the efforts intended to assist the population.

The review of related literature should be concisely summarized and should highlight key studies and findings. Articles reviewed should have been published within the last 7 years. Classic studies published more than 7 years ago can be reviewed and are the exception to the 7-year rule. If literature published in the last 7 years is lacking, authors should clearly identify this insufficiency. After concisely reviewing the literature, authors should help readers understand the gaps existing in the current literature and the need for the present study. See Chapter 3 for a more in-depth examination explaining the elements of various types of literature reviews.

Writing Exercises: Literature Review [commonly 2–3 double-spaced, typed pages]

- See Chapter 3 for more details about writing different types of literature reviews.
- Begin by reading the example papers at the end of the chapter to gain a clearer understanding of how to write a literature review for a needs assessment.
- Then go to the literature and complete a database search on your topic using key words. Identify all studies within a specified time period that directly relate to your topic.
- The literature review should synthesize the current published information regarding your topic so that readers can gain an understanding of what research has been completed to date.
- Generally, a synthesis means that you will summarize the existing literature using larger categories such as research design, specific population, sample size, findings, and limitations. It may be helpful for you to make a chart to organize this data so that you can present it in narrative form.
- When only a handful (≤5) of studies exist, authors may present more specific information about each of these studies instead of synthesizing them as a group.
- Literature reviews should end with a paragraph about what information is missing from the existing literature and how your study intends to fill this gap in the profession's knowledge base.
- Ask a peer who understands research methods and is familiar with your topic to read your literature review and provide feedback about its exhaustiveness and clarity.
- Make revisions based on the provided feedback.

Final Paragraph Before Methods [no heading needed]

The purpose statement is the final section after the Literature Review. Here, authors should state the purpose of the present needs assessment. A statement indicating that this knowledge may help occupational therapists to design effective intervention should follow. For example:

- The purpose of the present needs assessment was to determine the unique needs of parents with children with ASD who chronically refuse food. This knowledge may aid occupational therapists to better understand how to design effective intervention for this population.

- The purpose of the present needs assessment was to determine the unique needs of young adults with moderate intellectual disability who are attempting to transition from secondary to post-secondary education, employment, and life roles. This knowledge may aid occupational therapists to better understand how to design effective intervention for this population.
- The purpose of the present needs assessment was to determine the unique needs of children as their families are attempting to transition from shelter-living to supportive housing. This knowledge may aid occupational therapists to better understand how to design effective intervention for this population.

Note that when you write the final needs assessment paper, it is written in past tense.

Writing Exercises: Purpose Statement

- See the example papers at the end of this chapter for a clearer understanding of how to write a purpose statement for a needs assessment.
- Then practice writing a purpose statement for your capstone project.
- Begin with "The purpose of this needs assessment was to …" and complete the sentence with the primary objective of your project.
- Example: "The purpose of this needs assessment was to explore the experience of older adults who can no longer drive, but who need alternative methods to traverse the community."
- Remember that capstone projects are written in the past tense.

Definitions

All new and unfamiliar terms that are presented in the paper should be defined when the terms first appear. Common mistakes include failing to define terms, unclearly defining terms, presenting terms in one section and defining them in another, and changing the definition of a term throughout a paper.

Good definitions contain three elements (Mosey, 1996):

1. Label
2. Superordinate concept
3. Distinguishing characteristics

The label is the term used to describe a specific concept. The label chosen should be used consistently throughout the paper and should not change.

The superordinate concept is the larger umbrella term or category under which the term falls.

Distinguishing characteristics are the concepts that differentiate the term from similar concepts.

Examples of good definitions include the following:

- Repetitive strain disorders [label] are overuse syndromes [superordinate concept] in which the soft tissues of a joint become inflamed as a result of repeated engagement in activities that require continued movement [distinguishing concepts].

- Cognitive problem-solving strategies [label] are executive functions mediated by the frontal lobe [superordinate concept] that require the ability to identify a problem, plan a strategy, execute the strategy, evaluate the strategy's effect, and modify the strategy as needed [distinguishing characteristics].
- Food refusal [label] is the rejection of specific food types [superordinate concept] based on tastes, textures, consistencies, scents, and appearances that are aversive to the child [distinguishing concepts].

Writing Exercises: Definitions

- Make sure that all new and unfamiliar terms for readers are defined in your capstone project when they first appear. If you are unsure which terms may be new or unfamiliar to readers, ask a peer who does not know much about occupational therapy to read your work and identify such terms.
- Practice writing good definitions using the guidelines above and ensuring that you have a label, superordinate category, and distinguishing characteristics for all new and unfamiliar terms.
- To practice, define the term *occupational therapy*.
- Occupational therapy [label] is a health care profession [superordinate category] that assists people to restore or newly gain participation in desired daily life activities in home and community settings through skilled services, remediation, adaptation, and compensation [distinguishing characteristics].
- After writing several definitions, ask a peer to read them and let you know if they are clear. If they are not clear, ask the reader why or what part of the definition is unclear.
- Then revise the definitions with that feedback. Continue to use labels, superordinate categories, and distinguishing characteristics to structure your revised definitions.

Quotations

Quotations should only be used in scholarly writing when quoting a historical source or legal document; presenting a specific definition accepted by the scientific community, whose meaning would change if the exact wording was altered; and verbatim responses from patients or clients. Direct quotations of patient/client responses that were collected in a needs assessment are appropriate to present in the Results section. With the exception of these instances, quotations should be avoided in health care writing. Instead, paraphrase and cite the original source.

Method

The Method section of a needs assessment details your selection of a sample (from the larger population), collection of data (e.g., one-to-one interviews with 4 clients, a focus group with 6 clients, and an online questionnaire with 10 clients), and data analysis.

A concise and well-written Method section should be approximately 3–4 double-spaced, typed pages in length.

Needs Assessment Design

Needs Assessment Design is the first subheading in the Method section. The needs assessment design should be explained in this section. For example,

- Data for this needs assessment were collected through three 1-hour, one-to-one interviews with 4 clients.
- Data for this needs assessment were collected through an online questionnaire for adults attending a support group for parents with children exhibiting chronic food refusal.
- Data for this needs assessment were collected through two 1.5-hour focus groups of 6 seniors who stopped driving post-stroke and who presently report difficulty with desired community participation.

Writing Exercises: Needs Assessment Design [2–3 sentences]

- See the example papers at the end of this chapter for a clearer understanding of how to write the Needs Assessment Design section of your capstone project.
- Use the checklist at the end of this chapter to make an outline for the points that you want to make in your Needs Assessment Design section.
- Make sure to report the design that was used to collect data (e.g., one-to-one interviews, online questionnaire, in-person focus group).
- If institutional review board approval was obtained for the needs assessment to be carried out as a research study, indicate this here.
- Whether institutional review board approval was obtained or not, authors should obtain written consent from participants in the needs assessment to use their data in the capstone project.
- Ask a peer to read your Needs Assessment Design section and let you know if it is clear and contains all needed information. Make revisions as needed.

Participant Selection

Participant Selection is the second subheading in the Method section. Authors must describe the setting from which participants were selected to partake in the needs assessment. How did the author access participants and select those who would participate? What were the inclusion/exclusion criteria for participant selection?

Note that information about sample size and participant demographics should NOT be reported in this section. Instead, sample size and participant demographics are reported in the first paragraph of the Results.

Writing Exercises: Participant Selection [approximately 1 paragraph]

- See the example papers listed at the end of this chapter to gain a clearer understanding of how to write the Participant Selection section.
- Use the checklist at the end of this chapter to make an outline of your Participant Selection section.
- Make sure to describe how participants were accessed and from what setting they came.
- Provide the inclusion/exclusion criteria for participant selection.
- Ask a peer to read your Participant Selection section and describe who your targeted sample was, how they were accessed, from what setting(s) participants came, and what inclusion/exclusion criteria were used.
- If your reader could easily identify these, you have likely written a strong Participant Selection section. If they could not, revise your Participant Selection section using the above guidelines. Repeat the process of obtaining feedback and making revisions.

Instruments

Instruments is the third subheading in the Method section. The Instruments section will vary in length depending on the number of measures used.

- In a needs assessment, instruments will commonly be (a) an interview protocol of open-ended questions, (b) a focus group protocol of open-ended questions, or (c) a questionnaire.
- It is likely that these instruments will have been designed by the author for the present needs assessment, and thus, it is unlikely that any psychometric properties were established other than face validity using a panel of experts. Authors should document the instrument development process, stating that the instrument was developed specifically for the present needs assessment, and that, if relevant, only face validity was established by a panel of experts. The process of establishing face validity should be detailed.
- The instrument should be described with regard to number of questions, types of questions (open-ended, closed-ended, Likert scale items, or multiple-choice items), and administration length (time needed to complete the interview, focus group, or online questionnaire).
- The instrument questions should be provided in a figure or appendix.

Writing Exercises: Instruments [approximately 1–2 paragraphs]

- See the example papers listed at the end of this chapter to gain a clearer understanding of how to write the Instruments section.
- Use the checklist at the end of this chapter to make an outline of your Instruments section.

- Indicate what type(s) of instrument was used in the present needs assessment.
- If the instrument was designed by the author, state this clearly and describe the instrument development process. If face validity was established using a panel of experts, state this and describe the process.
- Describe the instrument with regard to the number of questions, types of questions, and length of administration.
- Ask a peer to review your Instruments section and describe the instrument and how it was developed. Ask them to identify what is clear and what is confusing.
- Use this feedback to make revisions. Once a second draft has been written, repeat the process of seeking feedback and making revisions with another peer.

Procedures

Procedures is the fourth subheading in the Method section. The Procedures section varies in length from 1 to 2 paragraphs.

The Procedures section documents the steps of the needs assessment after participants have been obtained. In other words, the steps of the interviews, focus group, or questionnaire are described in detail. For example,

> Each participant was interviewed in three separate, 1-hour interview sessions conducted by the author. Interviews took place in a private setting, such as the participant's home or a private office at the community center. All interviews were audio recorded and later transcribed by the author into a Word document. Interviews were scheduled at a time that was convenient for each participant and spaced over 2 months. A final fourth, 1-hour visit allowed the author to share her perceptions about participant data and seek verification from each participant. In this fourth visit, participants were able to confirm author perceptions or offer an alternate analysis.

Writing Exercises: Procedures [approximately 1–2 paragraphs]

- See the example papers listed at the end of this chapter to gain a clearer understanding of how to write the Procedures section.
- Then use the checklist at the end of this chapter to make an outline of your Procedures section.
- Using your outline, write the Procedures section of your Methods, making sure to document the steps of the needs assessment after participants have been obtained. In other words, the steps of the interviews, focus group, or questionnaire should be described in detail.
- Report the steps of the study in sufficient detail so that it can be evaluated and replicated by readers.

- Ask a peer to read your procedures section and describe it back to you, indicating what is clear and what needs greater clarification. Make revisions based on this feedback. Repeat the process of obtaining feedback and making revisions.

Data Collection

Data Collection is the subheading that directly follows the Procedures section. The Data Collection section is typically one paragraph. This section reports who collected data and the data collection schedule. For example,

> The author, an occupational therapist with 1 year of experience in the treatment of patients with adult ADHD, conducted the two focus groups. Focus groups took place 1 month apart so that the author could transcribe and review the first focus group session in order to prepare appropriate follow-up questions in the second focus group. The time frame of one month between focus group sessions was also chosen to provide participants with an opportunity to reflect upon questions and their answers, and to generate additional information. All focus groups were audio-recorded and transcribed by Quirkos Transcribe, which is a secure and encrypted automated transcription service.

Writing Exercises: Data Collection [approximately 1 paragraph]

- See the example papers listed at the end of this chapter to gain a clearer understanding of how to write the Data Collection section.
- Then use the checklist at the end of this chapter to make an outline of your Data Collection section.
- Using your outline, write the Data Collection section of your Methods making sure to document who collected data and the data collection schedule—in other words, when, where, and by whom data was collected in the Needs Assessment project.
- Also provide the name of software transcription programs or transcription services if used.
- Ask a peer to read your Data Collection section and describe it back to you, indicating what is clear and what needs greater clarification. Make revisions based on this feedback. Repeat the process of obtaining feedback and making revisions.

Data Analysis

Data Analysis is the subheading that directly follows *Data Collection*. The Data Analysis section is typically one paragraph. All descriptive (e.g., frequency counts, percentages) and qualitative data analysis methods used to analyze participant responses should be described and cited. For example,

Constant comparative analysis was used to analyze data in an iterative process in which interview transcripts were continuously coded and compared to identify themes and guide the direction of subsequent interviews. Constant comparative analysis was performed by the author after each interview and continued until no new themes could be generated (i.e., data saturation). This procedure was followed for each interview. Coding and theme development was based on a conventional content analysis approach (Creswell & Creswell, 2018; Hsieh & Shannon, 2005) in which small units of data are categorized first, followed by larger phrases and themes, and finally mega themes.

Writing Exercises: Data Analysis [approximately 1 paragraph]

- See the example papers listed at the end of this chapter to gain a clearer understanding of how to write the Data Collection section.
- Then use the checklist at the end of this chapter to make an outline of your Data Collection section.
- Using your outline, write the Data Collection section of your Methods, making sure to describe all descriptive and qualitative methods used to analyze your data.
- All data analysis methods should be based on accepted strategies documented in the literature and cited.
- If a software program was used to aid in data analysis, name and cite the software program.
- Document who participated in data analysis and what each person's role was.
- Ask a peer to read your Data Analysis section and describe it back to you, indicating what is clear and what needs greater clarification. Make revisions based on this feedback. Repeat the process of obtaining feedback and making revisions.

Results

The Results section directly follows the Data Analysis subheading and begins a new section of the manuscript. A concisely and well-written Results section should be approximately 2–4 double-spaced, typed pages in length. In the Results section, authors report their findings without interpreting them—interpretation of findings will be made in the Discussion section. The objective of the Results section is to report findings in a concise, clear, and sufficient way so that readers can verify reported results.

Begin the Results section with information about sample size and participant demographics. If participants began the needs assessment but then withdrew for various reasons, the number of participants who withdrew should be reported along with the reasons for withdrawal. Reporting standards require that age, gender, race, ethnicity, education level, socioeconomic status, and topic-specific characteristics such as functional status and community participation be provided for all participants in aggregate form (i.e., report the number followed by the percentage: n=8, 80%).

The qualitative data of the needs assessment should be organized by themes with supporting participant quotations. Quotations should be identified by participant number (each participant should be assigned a number, and their quotes should be accompanied by that identification), for example:

> When my child refuses five different foods in the span of 10 minutes, I feel powerless to help him and I'm scared for his survival.
>
> [Participant 3]

The Results section should consist of several themes gleaned from data analysis. Themes should serve as subheadings within the Results section, and each theme should be narratively described by the author and supported by 3–4 participant quotations.

Writing Exercises: Results [approximately 2–4 double-spaced, typed pages]

- See the example papers listed at the end of this chapter to gain a clearer understanding of how to write the Results section.
- Then use the checklist at the end of this chapter to make an outline of your Results section.
- Using your outline, write the Results section, making sure to provide findings without interpreting them (interpretation will be made in the Discussion section).
- Begin the Results section with information about sample size and participant demographics.
- Report whether any participants withdrew from participation and why (if known).
- The qualitative data of the needs assessment should be organized by themes with supporting participant quotations. Participants should be identified by a designated number.
- The Results section should be organized by the major themes that emerged through data analysis. Each theme should be narratively described by the author and supported by 3–4 participant quotations.
- Ask a peer to read your Results section and describe it back to you, indicating what is clear and what needs greater clarification. Make revisions based on this feedback. Repeat the process of obtaining feedback and making revisions.

Discussion

The Discussion section directly follows the Results and begins a new section of the paper. A concisely and well-written Discussion section should be approximately 3–4 double-spaced, typed pages in length.

Whereas the Results section is a reporting of the findings, the Discussion section in a needs assessment allows authors to interpret those findings as they relate to the sample and their experience of disability/dysfunction. Unanticipated findings should be addressed.

Authors should also attempt to discuss their findings in the context of what is known about the population through published literature. Are the findings congruent or inconsistent with published literature, and in what ways?

It is important that authors do not overstate their findings since the needs assessment is likely to have a small sample size. Findings can only be discussed with regard to that sample. While generalization of findings cannot be made, authors can suggest ways through which occupational therapists could address the clinical problems that were unearthed through the needs assessment in the sample's own clinical or community setting.

Writing Exercises: Discussion [approximately 3–4 double-spaced, typed pages]

- See the example papers listed at the end of this chapter to gain a clearer understanding of how to write the Discussion section.
- Then use the checklist at the end of this chapter to make an outline of your Discussion section.
- Using your outline, organize your Discussion section in accordance with the order of findings reported in the Results section. Each finding should be interpreted with regard to the specific sample that participated in the project and their experience of disability/dysfunction.
- Were any findings unexpected? If so, discuss the possible meaning of these findings and why they may have occurred.
- Authors should also discuss whether findings are novel or are congruent with previously reported literature.
- Make sure not to overstate your findings, as the needs assessment sample will likely be small and findings may not be able to be generalized to the larger population.
- Ask a peer to read your Discussion section and describe it back to you, indicating what is clear and what needs greater clarification. Make revisions based on this feedback. Repeat the process of obtaining feedback and making revisions.

Limitations

The Limitations section is a subsection of the Discussion and has its own subheading. The Limitations section is commonly 1–2 paragraphs.

A needs assessment has inherent weaknesses that should be documented in the Limitations section; the most common follow:

- Insufficient sample size negating generalization of findings to the larger population

- Sample selected from a convenience sample and from one geographical area of the country (both impeding generalization of findings to the larger population); the sample may not represent the larger population
- Possible influence of a Hawthorne effect (i.e., participants behaved differently than usual because they were aware that they were being interviewed or felt uncomfortable in the context of a focus group)

Writing Exercises: Limitations [1–2 paragraphs]

- See the example papers listed at the end of this chapter to gain a clearer understanding of how to write the Limitations section.
- Then use the checklist at the end of this chapter to make an outline of your Limitations section.
- Using your outline, write a draft of your Limitations section, noting the weaknesses in design.
- Ask a peer to read your Limitations section and describe it back to you, indicating what is clear and what needs greater clarification. Make revisions based on this feedback. Repeat the process of obtaining feedback and making revisions as needed.

Future Directions

If the needs assessment has not been carried out as a research study, the section following the Limitations is *Future Directions* (rather than *Future Research*, which is used when the needs assessment is a research study). The Future Directions section is approximately one paragraph.

Here, authors should identify (a) which questions remain unanswered and require further examination and (b) the direction for continued study. For example, if the needs assessment was completed with a small sample size and in one setting, authors could suggest that a future needs assessment be completed with a larger sample size and participants from a variety of settings.

Writing Exercises: Future Directions [approximately 1 paragraph]

- See the example papers listed at the end of this chapter to gain a clearer understanding of how to write the Future Directions section. Because these papers are research studies, the term *Future Research* was used.
- Then use the checklist at the end of this chapter to make an outline of your Future Directions section.
- Using your outline, write a draft of your Future Directions section, noting (a) the questions that continue to remain unanswered and require further examination, (b) next steps that should be taken to answer these questions, and (c) how the identified project limitations could be strengthened in a future project.

- Ask a peer to read your Future Directions section and describe it back to you, indicating what is clear and what needs greater clarification. Make revisions based on this feedback. Repeat the process of obtaining feedback and making revisions as needed.

Implications for Practice

The Implications for Practice section follows the Future Directions section and consists of approximately 6–8 bullets or one paragraph. Here, authors should cautiously describe how the findings of the needs assessment could be used. Because generalization of findings cannot be made beyond the present sample, authors can suggest ways through which the findings of their needs assessment can be used to help the participants in their own community or clinical setting.

Writing Exercises: Implications for Practice [approximately 6–8 bullets or 1 paragraph]

- See the example papers listed at the end of this chapter to gain a clearer understanding of how to write the Implications for Practice section. Note that because these papers are research studies, the Implications for Practice setting may have been generalized beyond the study sample.
- Then use the checklist at the end of this chapter to make an outline of your Implications for Practice section.
- Using your outline, write a draft of your Implications for Practice section. Note that your suggestions must pertain only to the participants in your needs assessment and cannot be generalized to the larger population. Describe how your findings can be translated into clinical practice that can help your participants with the needs that they identified. How can your findings be translated into occupational therapy practice that can help your participants enhance their performance of and participation in desired daily life activities in the home and community?
- Ask a peer to read your Implications for Practice section and describe it back to you, indicating what is clear and what needs greater clarification. Ask them to also provide feedback regarding whether your suggestions pertain only to your sample or extend beyond it to the larger population. If your suggestions have extended beyond your sample to the larger population, make revisions based on this feedback. Repeat the process of obtaining feedback and making revisions as needed.

Conclusion

In this final section of a needs assessment, authors should summarize the major findings and describe how these findings have potential to inform practice with the participants in their own communities.

The Conclusion section should be approximately one to two paragraphs.

Writing Exercises: Conclusion [approximately 1 paragraph]

- See the example papers listed at the end of this chapter to gain a clearer understanding of how to write the Conclusion section.
- Then use the checklist at the end of this chapter to make an outline of your Conclusion section.
- Using your outline, write a draft of your Conclusion section, making sure to (a) summarize the major findings of your needs assessment, (b) make suggestions about how to use your findings to provide occupational therapy services that help the participants to enhance their desired participation in daily life activities at home and in the community, and (c) identify questions that remain unanswered and outline the next steps that should be taken to answer these questions. Make sure not to generalize your statements beyond the participants in your needs assessment.
- Ask a peer to read your Conclusion section and describe it back to you, indicating what is clear and what needs greater clarification. Make revisions based on this feedback. Repeat the process of obtaining feedback and making revisions as needed.

After the Conclusion, the remaining manuscript sections in the order in which they should be presented are as follows:

- References
- Tables
- Figures

Checklist for Manuscript Structure and Content of Needs Assessments

Title

☐ Include the population's diagnosis/condition and age or developmental level.

☐ Indicate that the project was an examination of a population's needs; the words *needs assessment* (the design) should be inserted in the title.

Abstract

☐ Objectives: In 1–2 sentences, describe the purpose of the needs assessment. In a needs assessment, the purpose will address the systematic collection of data regarding a population's clinical needs in order to design intervention and inform future practice decisions.

☐ Method: In 1–2 sentences provide information about the population (diagnosis/condition, age group, functional status), sample size, needs assessment design (e.g., one-to-one interview, online questionnaire, focus group), and the setting from which patients/clients were selected.

☐ Results: In 1–2 sentences summarize findings about the sample's needs gleaned from data collection (interview, questionnaire, focus group).

☐ Conclusions: In 1–2 sentences describe the implications of the needs assessment findings with regard to how these preliminary findings can be used to inform practice in the sample's own clinical or community setting.

Introduction [no heading needed]

☐ Provide background information about the population and the problems they may encounter with regard to clinical course, function in daily life, and community participation.

☐ Background information relating to incidence or prevalence should also be provided.

☐ The implication of the population's problems, as they may impact the larger society, should be discussed.

☐ Indicate how the population's problems may be relevant to and *potentially* addressable by the profession.

☐ The need for the project should be made clear and answer the questions, "Why is this project needed now? What are the clinical needs of a population that traditionally does not receive occupational therapy services, but that could potentially benefit from them?"

Literature Review

☐ In a needs assessment, the literature review should focus on interventions that have been used by other professions to assist this population, the effectiveness of those interventions, and what is missing but needed by the population to attain optimal community participation.

☐ If no attempts to provide assistance to the population have been made by other professions, authors should clearly state this.

☐ Literature reviews should end with a paragraph about what information is missing from the existing literature and how your study intends to fill this gap in the profession's knowledge base.

Final Paragraph Before Methods [no heading needed]

☐ State the purpose of the present needs assessment.

☐ A statement indicating that this knowledge may help occupational therapists to design effective intervention for this population should follow.

Methods

Needs Assessment Design

☐ Report the design that was used to collect data (e.g., one-to-one interviews, online questionnaire, in-person focus group).

☐ If institutional review board approval was obtained for the needs assessment to be carried out as a research study, indicate this here.

☐ State that written consent was obtained from participants to use their data in the author's project.

Participant Selection

- ☐ Describe the setting from which participants were selected to partake in the needs assessment.
- ☐ Describe how participants were accessed and selected to participate.
- ☐ State the inclusion/exclusion criteria for participant selection.
- ☐ Note that information about sample size and participant demographics should NOT be reported in this section. This information is reported in the first paragraph of the Results.

Instruments

- ☐ Indicate what type(s) of instrument was used in the present needs assessment (e.g., an interview protocol of open-ended questions, a focus group protocol of open-ended questions, or a questionnaire).
- ☐ If the instrument was designed by the author, state this clearly and describe the instrument development process.
- ☐ If the instrument's face validity was established using a panel of experts, state this and describe the process.
- ☐ Describe the instrument with regard to number of questions, types of questions, and length of administration.
- ☐ Provide the instrument questions in a figure or appendix.

Procedures

- ☐ Document the steps describing how the needs assessment was carried out. In other words, document the steps of the interviews, focus groups, or questionnaires that were used with participants.
- ☐ Describe each step in detail so that another person can read about your project and replicate it.

Data Collection

- ☐ Document who collected data and the data collection schedule—in other words, when, where, and by whom data was collected in the needs assessment project.
- ☐ Also provide the name of software transcription programs or transcription services if used.

Data Analysis

- ☐ All descriptive (e.g., frequency counts, percentages) and qualitative data analysis methods used to analyze participant responses should be described and cited.
- ☐ If a software program was used to aid in data analysis, name and cite the software program.
- ☐ Document who participated in data analysis and what each person's role was.

Results

- ☐ Report findings without interpreting them; interpretation of findings will be made in the Discussion section.
- ☐ Begin the Results section with information about sample size and participant demographics (e.g., age, gender, race, ethnicity, education level, socioeconomic

status, and topic-specific characteristics such as functional status and community participation).

- ☐ Report whether any participants withdrew from participation and why (if known).
- ☐ Report all data in absolute numbers. If percentages are provided, they should accompany the absolute number from which the percentage was derived.
- ☐ The qualitative data of the needs assessment should be organized by themes with supporting participant quotations. Participants should be identified by a designated number.
- ☐ The Results section should be organized by the major themes that emerged through data analysis.
- ☐ Each theme should be narratively described by the author and supported by 3–4 participant quotations.

Discussion

- ☐ Organize your Discussion section in accordance with the order of findings reported in the Results section.
- ☐ Each finding should be interpreted with regard to the specific sample that participated in the study and their experience of disability/dysfunction. Interpretation should not extend beyond the project's sample.
- ☐ Authors should also attempt to discuss their findings in the context of what is known about the population through published literature. Are findings congruent or inconsistent with published literature, and in what ways?
- ☐ Did any unanticipated findings occur? Why may these have occurred?
- ☐ Make sure not to overstate findings, as the needs assessment sample will likely be small and findings may not be able to be generalized to the larger population.

Limitations

- ☐ Document the limitations of your needs assessment project. These may include any of the following:
    - ☐ Insufficient sample size negating generalization of findings to the larger population
    - ☐ Sample selected from a convenience sample and from one geographical area of the country (both impeding generalization of findings to the larger population); the sample may not represent the larger population
    - ☐ Possible influence of a Hawthorne effect (i.e., participants behaved differently than usual because they were aware that they were being interviewed or felt uncomfortable in the context of a focus group)

Future Directions

- ☐ Identify which questions remain unanswered and require further examination.
- ☐ Indicate the direction for continued study to address unanswered questions.
- ☐ Describe how the identified limitations could be strengthened in a future project.

Implications for Practice

- ☐ Describe how your findings can be translated into clinical practice that can help your participants with the needs that they identified.
- ☐ How can your findings be translated into occupational therapy practice that can help your participants enhance their performance of and participation in desired daily life activities in the home and community?

Conclusion

- ☐ Summarize the major findings of your needs assessment.
- ☐ Make suggestions about how to use your findings to provide occupational therapy services that could help the participants enhance their desired participation in daily life activities at home and in the community.
- ☐ Identify questions that remain unanswered and outline the next steps that should be taken to answer these questions.

Examples of Well-Written Needs Assessment Studies

Clymer, D. R., Fields, H. A., & Kniepmann, K. (2020). Assessing unmet needs of caregivers after stroke: Occupational therapist practices and perspectives. *Open Journal of Occupational Therapy, 8*(2), 1–13. https://doi.org/10.15453/2168-6408.1653

Gutman, S., Choi, A., Kearney, A., & Swarbrick, P. (2024). Understanding the needs of gender diverse youth and young adults and their staff members in homeless shelters and supported housing. *Open Journal of Occupational Therapy*, *2*(3), 1–17. https://doi.org/10.15453/2168-6408.2230

References

American Psychological Association. (2020). *Publication manual of the American Psychological Association* (7th ed.). Author.

Creswell, J. W., & Creswell, J. D. (2018). *Research design: Qualitative, quantitative, and mixed methods approaches* (5th ed.). SAGE.

Hsieh, H-F., & Shannon, S. E. (2005). Three approaches to qualitative content analysis. *Qualitative Health Research, 15*(9), 1277–1288. https://doi.org/10.1177/1049732305276687

Mosey, A. C. (1996). *Applied scientific inquiry in the health professions: An epistemological orientation* (2nd ed.). American Occupational Therapy Association.

CHAPTER 8

Manuscript Structure and Content for Case Reports and Case Series

A case report is a type of manuscript design in which the results of one patient's response to a novel intervention are reported, usually by the treating health care professional. A case series is similar to a case report but documents and compares the results of two or more patient responses to intervention. Case reports and case series were originally designed for physicians to describe the treatment and outcomes of one to three patients in response to a novel treatment method but have been adopted by other health care professionals. Traditional case reports and case series do not require the rigor of manualized intervention or written treatment guidelines (because treatment protocols are in the early stages of development), the use of instruments with established psychometric properties, baseline and postintervention measures, and statistical analysis of data. The CARE Guidelines (Gagnier et al., 2013; Rilet et al., 2017) provide a template and checklist for traditional case report and case series writing.

In the effort to build evidence supporting health care intervention methods, we recommend that case reports and case series be made more rigorous by the addition of preliminary written protocols, the use of instruments with strong psychometric properties, baseline and postintervention measures, basic statistical analysis of data when possible, and qualitative data describing the patient's(s') (or client's) perception of intervention. We additionally recommend that authors use the following structure and content for case report and case series writing.

Manuscript Headings and Formatting for Case Reports and Case Series

The following heading levels are based on American Psychological Association 7th edition (2020) formatting.

DOI: 10.4324/9781003734550-8

Title

Begin the manuscript with a title on a separate title page. The title should be centered, bolded, and typed in uppercase and lowercase letters.

Abstract

The Abstract should be placed on the page directly following the title page. The word *Abstract* should be capitalized, bolded, and centered. If keywords are required, they are inserted directly after the abstract and indented. The term *keywords* is italicized, capitalized, and indented:

Keywords: stroke, community participation, activities of daily living

Introduction

The Introduction begins on the page directly following the abstract. The heading *Introduction* is not typed in the manuscript because the beginning of the manuscript text alerts the reader that the Introduction has begun.

Literature Review

In capstone projects the Literature Review is commonly a separate section of the Introduction. In this case, the heading *Literature Review* is flush left, bolded, and capitalized. In published manuscripts the Literature Review may be a separate section of the Introduction or embedded in the Introduction without a heading.

Method

The Method section is positioned directly after the Introduction. The heading *Method* is centered, capitalized, and bolded.

Case Report Design or Case Series Design

Case Report Design, or Case Series Design, is the first subheading in the Method section. It is capitalized, bolded, and flush left.

Patient Selection and History

Patient Selection and History is the second subheading in the Method section. It is capitalized, bolded, and flush left.

Instruments (or Outcome Measures)

Instruments, or Outcome Measures, is the third subheading in the Method section. It is capitalized, bolded, and flush left.

Intervention

Intervention is the fourth subheading in the Method sections. It is capitalized, bolded, and flush left. In a case report or case series, two subheadings commonly fall under the heading *Intervention*: Intervention Description and Interveners.

Intervention Description

Intervention description is the first subheading of the Intervention section. It is a third-level heading that is italicized, capitalized, bolded, and flush left.

Interveners

Interveners, or Interventionists, is the second subheading of the Intervention section. It is a third-level heading that is italicized, capitalized, bolded, and flush left.

Data Collection

Data Collection is the subheading that directly follows Interveners. It is capitalized, bolded, and flush left.

Data Analysis

Data Analysis is the subheading that directly follows Data Collection. It is capitalized, bolded, and flush left.

Results

The Results section directly follows Data Analysis and begins a new section of the paper. The heading *Results* is capitalized, bolded, and centered.

Discussion

The Discussion section directly follows the Results section and begins a new section of the paper. The heading *Discussion* is bolded and centered.

Limitations

The Limitations subsection is part of the Discussion section but should be highlighted for the reader by a separate subheading within the Discussion section. The subheading *Limitations* is capitalized, bolded, and flush left.

Future Directions

The Future Directions section directly follows the Limitations subsection. This section is also part of the Discussion section and should be highlighted for the reader by a separate subheading label. The subheading *Future Directions* is capitalized, bolded, and flush left.

Implications for Practice

The Implications for Practice section follows the Future Directions section. The heading is capitalized, bolded, and flush left.

Conclusion

The Conclusion section follows the Implications for Practice section and is the final section in a capstone project paper and manuscript for publication. The heading is capitalized, bolded, and flush left.

References

References begin on a separate page following the Conclusion. The heading is centered, capitalized, and bolded.

Tables

Tables should be provided after the end of the references and begin on a separate page. Each table should be presented on its own page. Tables are named and presented in accordance with the order in which they are mentioned in the text. The title of the Table is inserted beneath the Table heading:

Table 1 [bolded, capitalized, and flush left]
Participant Demographics [italicized, capitalized, and flush left]

Figures

Figures should be provided after the end of the tables and begin on a separate page. Each figure should be presented on its own page. Figures are named and presented in accordance with the order in which they are mentioned in the text. The title of the Figure is inserted beneath the Figure heading:

Figure 1 [bolded, capitalized, and flush left]
Examples of Participant Quotes [italicized, capitalized, and flush left]

Manuscript Length

A case report or case series paper should be approximately 4,000 to 5,000 words in length. The length of a case report or case series should be shorter than a feature-length manuscript reporting an intervention effectiveness study. If authors intend to submit the paper for publication, they should refer to a specific journal's author guidelines to determine page length and word count for this type of manuscript.

Manuscript Heading Content for Case Reports and Case Series

There should be no repetition of content in the manuscript. The sections and subsections mentioned next should not contain overlap and will not if written as suggested.

Title

Case report and case series titles should contain four essential elements to help (a) readers understand the content and (b) indexers categorize the article so that it can be easily accessed by the intended audience.

- The patient's diagnosis and age group
- The intervention (the independent variable)
- The outcome measures (the dependent variable)
- The words *case report* or *case series* (the case design)

Examples of good case report titles include the following:

- Effect of a Social Skills Program on the Communication of a Nonverbal Adolescent with Autism: A Case Report
- Effect of Occupational Therapy Services on the Housing Transition of a Homeless Man with Psychiatric Disability and Substance Use: A Case Report
- A Case Report of Sensory Integration Therapy for a Child with Obsessive Compulsive Disorder

Examples of good case series titles include the following:

- Effect of a Social Skills Program on the Communication of Two Nonverbal Adolescents with Autism: A Case Series
- Effect of Occupational Therapy Services on the Housing Transition of Two Homeless Men with Psychiatric Disability and Substance Use: A Case Series
- A Case Series of Sensory Integration Therapy for Three Children with Obsessive Compulsive Disorder

Abbreviations in the title should be avoided unless commonly used and understood in the health care community.

Writing Exercises: Titles

- Practice writing a title for your case report or case series using the above guidelines and examples.
- Identify the patient's diagnosis or condition and age group, intervention, outcome measures, and case design (case report or case series) and combine these into one title.
- Ask a peer who does not know much about your project to read your title and tell you what they think your paper is about. If the reader is correct, you have likely written an adequate title. If they are not correct or are confused, you may need to revise your title using the above directions.

Abstract

Abstracts for case reports and case series are written similarly to those for intervention effectiveness studies and are best organized by use of the following headings, unless indicated otherwise by a specific journal's author guidelines: (a) objectives, (b) method, (c) results, and (d) conclusions. Addressing each subheading above—and the specific content that belongs in each subheading—will ensure that you provide readers, reviewers, and editors with essential information about the intervention, patient(s) or client(s), method, and findings. Because readers select papers primarily based on abstracts, the provision of this essential information is critical for the transparent reporting of case reports and case series. Although most case report and case series abstracts are between

150 and 200 words in length, authors are advised to check a specific journal's author guidelines and adhere to the stated word count.

- Objectives: In one to two sentences, authors should describe the purpose of the case. In a case report or case series, the purpose will address the initial assessment of a novel intervention for approximately 1–3 patients or clients.
- Method: In one to two sentences, authors should provide information about the patient(s) or client(s) (e.g., diagnosis or condition, age group, functional status), setting, case design (e.g., case report with pre- and posttest measures), intervention length and description, follow-up points if any, and outcome measures.
- Results: In one to two sentences, authors should report findings about the intervention's effect (if used, statistical test results, p values, and confidence intervals should be reported) and the patient's (or patients') perceptions of intervention.
- Conclusions: In one to two sentences, authors should (a) describe the implications of the intervention for the patient's (or patients') functional status and independence and (b) address how these preliminary findings can be used to inform future research and practice.

Writing Exercises: Abstract [approximately 150–200 words]

- See the example papers at the end of this chapter to gain a clearer understanding of how to write an abstract for a case report or case series.
- The abstract is the last section that should be written after all other manuscript sections are completed.
- Practice writing an abstract for your manuscript using the provided guidelines.
- Objectives: Go to the purpose statement of your manuscript and identify the purpose of the paper. Modify this sentences(s) so that it is not taken verbatim from the manuscript text.
- Method: Go to your Methods section of your manuscript and identify information regarding the following: participants (e.g., number of patients, diagnosis or condition, selection strategy), case report or case series design, intervention, and data collection procedures. Revise these sentences so that they are not written verbatim and can be shortened and combined into one to two sentences.
- Results: Select the primary findings from your Results section. You will likely not be able to report all of your findings in the abstract. Select approximately two primary results that are most salient to your manuscript. Try to rewrite these sentences so that they are shortened into one to two sentences. If statistical analysis was used, each result should be accompanied by the statistical test result, exact p value, and confidence interval.
- Conclusions: Go to your Discussion section and select one to two primary points regarding the implications of your findings for future research and clinical practice development. Rewrite these sentences so that they are shortened into one to two sentences.

- If you are submitting this manuscript for publication, check to ensure that the word count is within the required limitations of the journal to which you are submitting. If needed, go back through all abstract sections and reduce word length.
- Ask a peer, who ideally is a health care professional, to read your abstract and let you know if it is clear, and if not, what can be made clearer.

Introduction [no heading needed]

The Introduction of a case report or case series should be no longer than four double-spaced, typed pages. Similar to intervention effectiveness studies, the Introduction of case reports and case series should provide background information about the problem as it relates to the patient (or client), profession, and society. Information about the patient diagnosis or condition (relating to incidence and functional independence in the community) should be provided. The need for the novel intervention examined in the present paper should be justified for the reader and the intervention should be briefly described; a detailed description of the intervention will be provided in the Method section. Authors should also discuss the theoretical basis for the novel intervention.

Writing Exercises: Introduction

- See the example papers at the end of this chapter to understand how to write clear Introduction sections.

Background [approximately 2–3 paragraphs]

- Practice writing the Introduction section of your manuscript. Begin by describing the background of the problem as it relates to your specific patients (or clients). Most backgrounds begin with information about prevalence or incidence rate of the addressed clinical condition.
- Describe the current problem with regard to the patient's (patients') daily life function, community participation, or some other important aspect of their life situation. Have the patients received previous intervention and what was the effectiveness of the intervention?

Need Section [commonly 2 paragraphs]

- The need section in a case report or case series relates to the need to develop and assess a novel intervention for a specific patient or small group of patients because previous intervention either did not exist or has not been effective.
- Once you have drafted the background and need statement, ask a peer (ideally a health care professional) to read your work and describe the background and need for your intervention. If the reader could not adequately describe the

background and need as you intended, identify what they missed and rewrite those components.

- Once you have revised the background and need statement, repeat this last step with another peer, ideally a health care professional, who is unfamiliar with your work.

Writing Exercises: Description of the Intervention [approximately 1–2 paragraphs]

- When an intervention is novel, authors should provide a description of the intervention, its theoretical base, and proposed methods of delivery.
- See the example papers at the end of this chapter to understand how to write a clear description of the intervention within the Introduction.
- Authors should state that they developed this novel intervention to meet a treatment need that was lacking for a specific clinical population.
- Describe the theoretical bases that were used to develop the intervention.
- Include a description of the intervention's intended delivery methods (e.g., one-to-one therapy, group therapy, video instruction, virtual visits).
- Do not describe details such as overall length of intervention, number of sessions per week, and length of each session, or what is typically referred to as dosage and duration. These details will be placed in the Method section.

A concise and well-written Introduction should be approximately three to four double-spaced, typed pages in length.

Literature Review

In a case report or case series, the literature review should describe the interventions that have traditionally been used for your patient's (or patients') diagnosis or condition. Information about the effectiveness of these interventions should be assessed for the reader. If your intervention is a novel one within the profession of occupational therapy, describe the occupational therapy interventions that have traditionally been used with this clinical population along with their effectiveness. If previous interventions have never been provided to this clinical population by occupational therapists, describe interventions used by other professions, such as psychologists, nurses, and behaviorists. The literature review should justify why your novel intervention is needed. The 7-year rule for citation use should be applied; however, when more recent literature does not exist, articles with publication dates of more than 7 years can be used to discuss the theoretical base, traditionally used interventions for this diagnosis, and studies of similar treatment approaches. Articles about incidence should not be older than 2 to 3 years.

Writing Exercises: Literature Review [commonly 2–3 double-spaced, typed pages]

- See Chapter 3 for more details about writing different types of literature reviews.
- Begin by reading the example papers at the end of the chapter to gain a clearer understanding of how to write literature reviews.
- Then go to the literature and complete a database search on your patient's (or patients') clinical condition and traditionally used interventions. Identify all studies within a specified time period that directly relate to your target population and novel intervention.
- The literature review should synthesize the current published information so that readers can gain an understanding of what research has been completed to date and what may be lacking.
- Generally, a synthesis means that you will summarize the existing literature using larger categories such as research design, specific population, sample size, and findings. It may be helpful for you to make a chart to organize this data so that you can present it in narrative form.
- When only a handful (≤5) of intervention studies exist, authors may present more specific information about each of these studies instead of synthesizing them as a group.
- Literature reviews should end with a paragraph about what information is missing from the existing literature and how your study intends to fill this gap in the profession's knowledge base.
- Ask a peer, ideally a health care professional, to read your literature review and provide feedback about its exhaustiveness and clarity.
- Make revisions based on the provided feedback.

Final Paragraph Before Methods [no heading needed]
The purpose statement is the final paragraph before the Methods. Here, authors should state the purpose of the present case report or case series.

- The purpose of the present case series was to determine if a client-centered, sensory based nutritional diet can decrease food refusal in three children with autism spectrum disorder.
- The purpose of the present case series was to determine if a robotic device can increase upper extremity use in two adults with hemiplegia 1-month post stroke.
- The purpose of the present case report was to determine if a housing and life skills program can help a homeless man to transition from a shelter to supportive housing and maintain housing at 6-month follow-up.

Case questions should contain the patient diagnosis/condition and age group, intervention, and outcome measures. Case questions should clearly indicate that the case design involves one to three patients (or clients). Case questions generally relate to effectiveness, dosage and duration, and patient (or client) satisfaction and tolerance. If case questions were not formally developed at the outset of treatment, authors can discuss the clinical hypotheses that supported their decision to develop and administer intervention.

Examples of good case report and case series questions include the following:

- Can a 10-week client-centered, sensory-based, nutritional diet decrease food refusal in a child with autism spectrum disorder?
- Can two adults with hemiplegia 1-month post stroke tolerate a 4-hour-per-day robotic training program to increase upper extremity use?
- What are client perceptions of a housing and life skills program designed to help three homeless men transition from a shelter to supportive housing and maintain housing at 6-month follow-up?

Writing Exercises: Purpose Statement

- See the example papers at the end of this chapter for a clearer understanding of how to write a purpose statement.
- Then practice writing a purpose statement for your case report or case series.
- Begin with "The purpose of the present case report (or case series) was to ..." and complete the sentence with the primary objective of your project.
- Example: "The purpose of the present case report was to assess the effectiveness of a novel lymphedema reduction movement program for a woman with lymphedema secondary to mastectomy."
- Remember that all case reports and case series are written in the past tense.

Writing Exercises: Case Questions

- See the example papers listed at the end of this chapter for a clearer understanding of how to write case questions.
- Practice writing case questions for your project using the provided guidelines.
- Make sure to include the target population, intervention, case design, and outcome measures.
- Remember that case questions generally address effectiveness, dosage and duration, and patient (or client) satisfaction and tolerance.
- Ask a peer to read your case questions and then explain what you are seeking through your project. If the reader is accurate, you have likely written good case questions. If they are not accurate, revise your case questions based on the strategies outlined above. Repeat the process of seeking feedback and making revisions.

Definitions

All new and unfamiliar terms that are presented in the Introduction (and throughout the text) should be defined when the term first appears in the manuscript. Common mistakes include failing to define terms, unclearly defining terms, presenting terms in one section and defining them in another, and changing the definition of a term within a paper.

Good definitions contain three elements (Mosey, 1996):

1. Label
2. Superordinate concept
3. Distinguishing characteristics

The label is the term used to describe a specific concept. The label chosen should be used consistently throughout the paper and should not change.

The superordinate concept is the larger umbrella term or category under which the term falls.

Distinguishing characteristics are the concepts that differentiate the term from similar concepts.

Examples of good definitions include the following:

- Repetitive strain disorders [label] are overuse syndromes [superordinate concept] in which the soft tissues of a joint become inflamed as a result of repeated engagement in activities that require continued movement [distinguishing concepts].
- Cognitive problem-solving strategies [label] are executive functions mediated by the frontal lobe [superordinate concept] that require the ability to identify a problem, plan a strategy, execute the strategy, evaluate the strategy's effect, and modify the strategy as needed [distinguishing characteristics].
- Food refusal [label] is the rejection of specific food types [superordinate concept] based on tastes, textures, consistencies, scents, and appearances that are aversive to the child [distinguishing concepts].

Writing Exercises: Definitions

- Make sure that all new and unfamiliar terms for readers are defined in your manuscript when they first appear. If you are unsure about which terms may be new or unfamiliar to readers, ask a peer to read your work and identify such terms.
- Practice writing good definitions using the guidelines above and ensuring that you have a label, superordinate category, and distinguishing characteristics for all new and unfamiliar terms.
- To practice, define the term *occupational therapy*.
- Occupational therapy [label] is a health care profession [superordinate category] that assists people to restore or newly gain participation in desired daily life

activities in home and community settings through skilled services, remediation, adaptation, and compensation [distinguishing characteristics].

- After writing several definitions, ask a peer to read them and let you know if they are clear. If they are not clear, ask the reader why or what part of the definition is unclear.
- Then revise the definitions with that feedback. Continue to use labels, superordinate categories, and distinguishing characteristics to structure your revised definitions. Repeat the process of seeking feedback and making revisions.

Quotations

Quotations should only be used in scholarly writing when quoting a historical source or legal document; presenting a specific definition accepted by the scientific community, whose meaning would change if the exact wording was altered; and verbatim responses from patients or clients. With the exception of these instances, quotations should be avoided in health care writing. Instead, paraphrase and cite the original source. In case reports and case series, it is acceptable to provide direct quotes of patient/client responses.

Method

The Method section of case reports and case series details your selection of a patient or client for the novel intervention, collection of baseline measures, intervention administration, collection of posttest measures, and analysis of findings. The Method section must provide specific details about the above so that (a) researchers can replicate findings and design larger studies; (b) practitioners can determine if the intervention may have potential benefit for their own patients; and (c) editors, reviewers, and readers can evaluate the rigor of the case methodology. The use of the following subheadings in the Method section, and the content belonging in each subheading, will help you provide transparent and essential information.

Case Report Design [or Case Series Design]

The case design, or the sequence of treatment and data collection, should be explained in this section. For example:

- Pretest/posttest design with 3-month follow-up
- Baseline data collection, first intervention period, first postintervention data collection, second intervention period, second postintervention data collection

In addition to the sequence of treatment and data collection, authors should indicate that patients provided consent for their data to be used in a capstone project or future publication (authors should ethically obtain patient consent once the decision has been made to use patient data for a case report or case series). If at some point, authors wish to publish their case report or case series, they should obtain institutional review board or ethics committee approval retrospectively.

Writing Exercises: Case Report Design or **Case Series Design** [approximately 1 paragraph]

- See the example papers listed at the end of this chapter for a clearer understanding of how to write the Case Design subsection for a case report or case series.
- Use the checklist at the end of this chapter to make an outline of your Case Design section.
- Write the Case Design section of your Methods making sure to
  - Thoroughly describe the case design.
  - State that informed consent was obtained from adult patients or assent from child patients (or both when appropriate).
  - If authors intend to publish findings, indicate that institutional review board or ethics committee approval was obtained retrospectively.
- Ask a peer, ideally a health care professional, to read your Case Report or Case Series Design section and let you know if it is clear and contains all needed information. Use this feedback to make revisions and repeat the process of obtaining feedback and making revisions.

Patient Selection and History

Authors must describe the setting from which the patient(s) was selected to receive the novel treatment, the patient characteristics that designated them as a good candidate for the novel intervention, and the patient's (or patients') health history. Minimal reporting standards require that patient demographics include age, gender, race, ethnicity, and socioeconomic status. Functional status and level of independence in community participation should also be addressed. Transparent reporting standards require that the healthcare professional who selected the patient for intervention, and the relationship of that person to the patient, be disclosed in this section.

Writing Exercises: Patient Selection and History [approximately 1–2 paragraphs]

- See the example papers listed at the end of this chapter for a clearer understanding of how to write the Patient Selection and History subsection for a case report or case series.
- Use the checklist at the end of this chapter to make an outline of your Patient Selection and History section.
- Write the Patient Selection and History section of your Methods making sure to
  - Report patient demographics.
  - Report functional status and level of independence in community participation.
  - Indicate the patient characteristics that designated the patient(s) as a good candidate for the novel intervention.
  - Describe the setting from which the patient(s) was selected.

  - Disclose the relationship between the treating health professional and the patient.
- Ask a peer, ideally a health care professional, to read your Patient Selection and History section and let you know if it is clear and contains all needed information. Use this feedback to make revisions and repeat the process of obtaining feedback and making revisions until complete.

Instruments [or Outcome Measures]

All instruments and outcome measures (such as frequency counts of specific behaviors) used to gather baseline and postintervention data should be described and cited in this section. Detailed descriptions of all instruments will allow readers to evaluate whether the selected instruments were appropriate to measure the targeted outcomes. Instruments (including clinical assessment tools such as goniometers, edema volumeters, and dynamometers) should be described with regard to purpose, intended population, type of data collected (e.g., self-report, performance-based observer rating, Likert scale, open-ended questions, or total score yielding ratio data), and administration length. Psychometric properties of each instrument should be provided in numeric value, with statistical test results, *p* values, and confidence intervals indicated (all psychometric properties should be cited). If authors have used an instrument without established psychometric properties or if an instrument has been newly developed for this case report or case series, this information must be clearly stated in this section. Using instruments without established reliability and validity may yield questionable findings, and authors should justify their decision to use such an instrument. Frequency counts of desired behaviors (or other clinically targeted outcomes), however, do not require reliability and validity data and are appropriate for case reports and case series. If authors have developed an assessment for this case report or case series to measure a specific outcome, they should describe the development process and disclose if procedures included the evaluation of face or content validity through an expert panel. The provision of sample items in a table or figure will help readers understand whether the newly developed instrument targets the examined outcome measure for which it was designed.

Writing Exercises: Instruments or **Outcome Measures** [approximately 3–4 paragraphs depending on number of instruments]

- See the example papers listed at the end of this chapter for a clearer understanding of how to write the Instruments (or Outcomes) subsection for a case report or case series.
- Use the checklist at the end of this chapter to make an outline of your Instruments section.
- Write the Instruments section of your Methods making sure to

- Describe and cite all instruments and outcome measures (such as frequency counts of specific behaviors) used to gather baseline and postintervention data.
- Provide the psychometric properties of each instrument in numeric value, with statistical test results, *p* values, and confidence intervals indicated.
- Indicate whether any instruments do not have established psychometric properties or were developed specifically for this case report or case series.
- If instruments were developed specifically for this case report or case series, describe the process of development and indicate whether face validity was established by a panel of experts. Provide sample items in a table.
- Frequency counts of desired behaviors (or other clinically targeted outcomes) do not require reliability and validity data and are appropriate for case reports and case series.

- Ask a peer, ideally a health care professional, to read your Instruments (or Outcomes) section and let you know if it is clear and contains all needed information. Use this feedback to make revisions and repeat the process of obtaining feedback and making revisions until complete.

Intervention

The Intervention section for case reports and case series is divided into the following two subsections:

Intervention Description

The intervention should be described with regard to the following:

- The number and length of sessions (dosage) and the length of the intervention over time (duration)
- The content and setting of each session
- Whether intervention was delivered individually or in a group, and in-person or virtually

The clinical course should be described including any interruption in or discontinuation of treatment. Authors should disclose whether the patient received any type of simultaneous clinical service that could not be controlled and whose influence may have affected results.

Interveners [or Interventionists]

Information about those providing intervention should detail the following:

- The type of professional(s) who provided treatment
- The number of therapists involved in care
- The type and length of training that the therapist(s) received to administer intervention

In case reports and case series, it is common for one therapist to provide all care; however, if more than one therapist provided care, authors should describe the procedures to ensure that all interveners provided intervention uniformly.

Writing Exercises: Intervention [approximately 2–4 paragraphs]

- See the example papers listed at the end of this chapter for a clearer understanding of how to write the Intervention section for a case report or case series.
- Use the checklist at the end of this chapter to make an outline of your Intervention section.
- Make sure to address the following:
  - Intervention Description
    - Describe the intervention with regard to
      - The number and length of sessions (dosage) and the length of the intervention over time (duration)
      - The content and setting of each session
      - Whether intervention was delivered individually or in a group, and in-person or virtually
      - The occurrence of any interruption in or discontinuation of treatment (and why that occurred)
      - Whether patients received any simultaneous treatment that may have influenced outcomes
  - Interveners
    - Describe interveners with regard to
      - The type of professional(s) who provided treatment
      - The number of therapists involved in care
      - The type and length of training that the therapist(s) received to administer intervention
      - If more than one therapist provided care, authors should describe the procedures to ensure that all interveners provided intervention uniformly.
- Ask a peer, ideally a health care professional, to read your Intervention section and let you know if it is clear and contains all needed information. Ask the person to identify what is missing or confusing. Use this feedback to make revisions.

Data Collection

In a case report or case series, it is common for the treating therapist to collect data; however, such overlap of roles should be clearly stated because this condition may introduce bias and influence results. Authors should describe how, when, and by whom each set of data was collected. If multiple data collectors were used, authors should detail how data collectors were trained to collect data uniformly and whether interrater reliability was established.

Writing Exercises: Data Collection [approximately 1–3 paragraphs]

- See the example papers listed at the end of this chapter for a clearer understanding of how to write the Data Collection section for a case report or case series.
- Use the checklist at the end of this chapter to make an outline of your Data Collection section.
- Make sure to address the following:
  - Describe how, when, and by whom each set of data was collected.
  - Disclose whether the treating therapist also collected data. This situation is common in case designs but should be disclosed because of the possible bias that may influence findings.
  - If more than one data collector was used, describe how data collectors were trained to collect data uniformly and whether interrater reliability was established among data collectors.
- Ask a peer, ideally a health care professional, to read your Data Collection section and let you know if it is clear and contains all needed information. Ask the person to identify what is missing or confusing. Use this feedback to make revisions.

Data Analysis

All descriptive, statistical, and qualitative data analysis methods used to compare baseline and postintervention measures and analyze the patient's perceptions of treatment should be described and cited. Statistical analysis that will likely be unfamiliar to readers or is incongruent with traditional parametric and nonparametric data analysis rules should be justified and cited. Similarly, descriptive and qualitative methods used to understand the patient's response to treatment should be described and cited. The names and citations of all analytic software programs should also be provided, and the level at which statistical significance was set for quantitative tests should be reported.

Writing Exercises: Data Analysis [approximately 2 paragraphs]

- See the example papers listed at the end of this chapter for a clearer understanding of how to write the Data Analysis section for a case report or case series.
- Use the checklist at the end of this chapter to make an outline of your Data Analysis section.
- Make sure to address the following:
  - Describe and cite all descriptive, statistical, and qualitative data analysis methods used to compare baseline and postintervention measures.
  - Indicate at what statistical level probability was set.

- Describe and cite all qualitative data analysis methods used to understand patient satisfaction and perceptions of intervention.
- Name and cite all software programs used in data analysis.

- Ask a peer, ideally a health care professional, to read your Data Analysis section and let you know if it is clear and contains all needed information. Ask the person to identify what is missing or confusing. Use this feedback to make revisions.

A concisely and well-written Method section should be approximately three to four double-spaced, typed pages in length.

Results

The Results section in a case report or case series (a) details the findings of baseline, postintervention, and follow-up measures; and (b) documents the patient's perception of intervention through self-report measures and qualitative interviews. The patient's intervention experience should include information about satisfaction, congruence with cultural values, and ability to help the patient attain personal health goals. Family member and caregiver reports may also be used to provide supplemental information in addition to the patient's responses, particularly when patients may experience cognitive disorders that limit or alter perception or when children are participants. Authors should aim to supplement quantitative and qualitative data with information about gains the patient has made in postintervention functional community participation based on patient, family member, caregiver, and teacher, etc., reports. The Results section should be organized in accordance with the order of case questions outlined in the purpose statement. Findings should be reported for each case question. While the provision of raw scores is not typical in intervention effectiveness studies with multiple participants, raw score reporting in tables and figures is customary in case reports and case series. When statistical analysis has been performed to compare baseline and postintervention measures, the statistical test results, *p* values, and confidence intervals should be reported. Qualitative data may be supported by quotations from the patient, family member, or caregiver. Authors should also document the occurrence of any adverse effects or unexpected findings.

See Chapter 10, Reporting Statistical Data in Text and Tables, to clarify how to correctly report statistical tests and symbols in the Results section.

A concisely and well-written Results section should be approximately three to four double-spaced, typed pages in length.

Writing Exercises: Results [approximately 3–4 doubled-spaced, typed pages]

- See the example papers listed at the end of this chapter for a clearer understanding of how to write the Results section for a case report or case series.
- Use the checklist at the end of this chapter to make an outline of your Results section.

- Make sure to address the following:
  - Organize your Results section in accordance with the order of case questions in your purpose statement. Report findings for each case question.
  - Report findings for all baseline, postintervention, and follow-up measures for each patient.
  - Report findings about the patient's perception of intervention gained through self-report measures and/or qualitative interviews. Findings should pertain to the patient's satisfaction with the intervention, the intervention's congruence with their cultural values, and the intervention's ability to help the patient attain personal health goals.
  - Family member and caregiver reports may also be used to provide supplemental information about the intervention's perceived effect.
  - Supplemental information should focus on the intervention's impact on the patient's postintervention functional community participation.
  - Document the occurrence of any adverse effects or unexpected findings.
- Ask a peer, ideally a health care professional, to read your Results section and let you know if it is clear and contains all needed information. Ask the person to identify what is missing or confusing. Use this feedback to make revisions.

Discussion

The Discussion section in a case report or case series allows authors to interpret the findings reported in the Results section as they relate to the patient. It is important that authors do not overstate their findings about the intervention's effectiveness because case reports and case series lack the rigor of control, randomization, larger sample sizes, and anonymization procedures. In a case report and case series, authors can only state that the intervention appeared to be effective with the participating patient. While generalization of findings cannot be made, authors can suggest that the intervention shows promise and warrants future study with larger sample sizes and more rigorous study methods. The Discussion section should be organized according to the order of case questions provided in the purpose statement and addressed in the Results section. Authors should attempt to answer each case question based on findings presented in the Results section. Unanticipated findings should be explained, and the occurrence of adverse events should be examined with regard to intervention risk and safety. Authors should discuss how the case report/case series findings can inform future research needed to build consensus regarding best practice.

Writing Exercises: Discussion [approximately 4–5 doubled-spaced, typed pages]

- See the example papers listed at the end of this chapter for a clearer understanding of how to write the Discussion section for a case report or case series.
- Use the checklist at the end of this chapter to make an outline of your Discussion section.

- Make sure to address the following:
  - Organize your Discussion section in accordance with the order of case questions in your purpose statement. Interpret the findings for each case question.
  - Attempt to explain findings for all baseline, postintervention, and follow-up measures for each patient.
  - Explain all unanticipated findings and the occurrence of adverse events as they relate to intervention risk and safety.
  - In a case report and case series, authors can only state that the intervention appeared to be effective with the participating patient(s) due to lack of control, randomization, larger sample sizes, and anonymization procedures. It is important not to overstate findings.
  - Although generalization of the findings from case reports and case series cannot be made to the larger population, authors can suggest that the intervention shows promise and warrants future study with larger sample sizes and more rigorous study methods.
  - Suggest how the case report/case series findings can inform future research needed to build consensus regarding best practice.
- Ask a peer, ideally a health care professional, to read your Discussion section and let you know if it is clear and contains all needed information. Ask the person to identify what is missing or confusing. Use this feedback to make revisions.

Limitations

Case reports and case series have inherent weaknesses in internal and external validity that should be documented in the Limitations section.

Weaknesses in internal validity (i.e., the degree to which researchers can be confident that the changes in outcome measures were a result of the intervention) include the following:

- Possible lack of intervention fidelity if multiple interveners were used
- Compromised anonymization of the intervener(s) and data collector(s) if intervention was provided by the same therapist who collected data
- Insufficient sample size power
- Lack of control and randomization
- Possible use of instruments with little or no established psychometric properties

Weaknesses in external validity (i.e., the degree to which researchers can be confident that the participants represent the larger population) include the following:

- Possible influence of participant incentives on case findings
- One to three patient findings cannot be generalized to the larger population

If follow-up points were not incorporated into the case report/case series design, a further weakness would involve the inability to understand whether gains made as a possible result of intervention lasted over time.

Writing Exercises: Limitations [approximately 1 paragraph]

- See the example papers listed at the end of this chapter for a clearer understanding of how to write the Limitations section for a case report or case series.
- Use the checklist at the end of this chapter to make an outline of your Limitations section.
- Determine if any of the following weaknesses apply to your case and should be documented in the Limitations section:
  - If multiple interveners were used, there may be a possible lack of intervention fidelity
  - Potential bias if intervention and data collection were carried out by the same therapist
  - Insufficient sample size power
  - Lack of control and randomization
  - Possible use of instruments with little or no established psychometric properties
  - Participant incentives may have biased findings
  - Generalization cannot be made from 1–3 patients to the larger population
  - If follow-up points were not built into the case design, it is difficult to understand if patient gains resulting from intervention were maintained over time.
- Ask a peer, ideally a health care professional, to read your Discussion section and let you know if it is clear and contains all needed information. Ask the person to identify what is missing or confusing. Use this feedback to make revisions.

Future Directions

In the Future Directions section, authors can recommend future study designs that address the previously noted limitations. This section is approximately one paragraph.

Implications for Practice

Implications for Practice can only relate to the patient(s) in the case and their own clinical course over time, how findings can be used to design future research with more rigorous methodologies, and how findings from the case can be used to begin to build clinical consensus about practice decisions. This section is approximately one paragraph or 4–6 bullets.

Conclusion

In this final section of a case report or case series, authors should summarize the major case findings and describe how these findings have potential to inform future research that can build consensus about practice decisions.

A concisely and well-written Discussion section should be approximately four to five double-spaced, typed pages in length.

After the end of the Discussion section, the following are the remaining manuscript sections in the order in which they should be presented in the paper:

- References
- Tables
- Figures

Checklist for Manuscript Structure and Content of Case Reports and Case Series

Title

☐ Include the following elements: patient diagnosis and age group, intervention, outcome measures, and case report or case series.

Abstract

☐ Objectives: In one to two sentences, describe the purpose of the case project. In a case report or case series, the purpose will address the initial assessment of a novel intervention for a specific patient (or client) or small group of one to three patients.

☐ Method: In one to two sentences, provide information about the patient(s) or client(s) (e.g., diagnosis/condition, age group, functional status), setting, case design (e.g., case report with pre- and posttest measures), intervention length and description, follow-up points if any, and outcome measures.

☐ Results: In one to two sentences, report findings about the intervention's effect (if used, statistical test results, *p* values, and confidence intervals should be reported) and the patient's (or patients') perceptions of intervention.

☐ Conclusions: In one to two sentences, (a) describe the implications of the intervention for the patient's functional status and independence and (b) address how these preliminary findings can be used to inform future research and practice.

Introduction

☐ Provide background information about the problem as it relates to the patient(s), profession, and society.

☐ Provide information about the patient diagnosis or condition relating to incidence and functional independence in the community.

☐ Briefly describe the novel intervention.

☐ Discuss the intervention's theoretical base.

Literature Review

☐ Discuss traditional interventions (and their effectiveness) used to address the problems associated with the diagnosis or condition.

☐ Justify the need for the novel intervention.

Final Paragraph Before Methods

☐ Purpose statement: state the purpose of the present case report or case series.

- ☐ Case questions: provide clear and precise case questions that contain patient diagnosis/condition and age group, intervention, and outcome measures. Indicate that only one to three patients are involved.
- ☐ Case questions generally relate to effectiveness, dosage and duration, and patient (or client) satisfaction and tolerance.
- ☐ If case questions were not formally developed at the outset of treatment, discuss clinical hypotheses.
- ☐ Make sure that all terms are well defined as soon as they are presented in the manuscript.

Method

Case Report Design or Case Series Design

- ☐ Describe the case design or sequence of treatment and data collection.
- ☐ Indicate that patient consent was obtained.
- ☐ Indicate whether institutional review board or ethics committee approval was obtained.

Patient Selection and History

- ☐ Describe the setting from which the patient was selected, patient characteristics, and patient health history.
- ☐ Describe patient demographics including age, gender, race, ethnicity, and socioeconomic status.
- ☐ Describe functional status and level of independence in community participation.
- ☐ Identify the person who selected the patient for intervention and that person's relationship to the patient.

Instruments (or Outcome Measures)

- ☐ Describe and cite all instruments and outcome measures used to gather baseline and postintervention data regarding purpose, intended population, type of data collected, and administration length.
- ☐ Provide the psychometric properties for each instrument in numeric value, with statistical test results, p values, and confidence intervals indicated; provide citations for all established psychometric properties. Disclose if no established psychometric properties exist.
- ☐ If an assessment has been newly developed for this case report or case series, describe the development process. Provide sample items in a table or figure.

Intervention

Intervention Description

- ☐ Describe the number and length of sessions (dosage); the length of the intervention over time (duration); the content of each session; and whether intervention was delivered individually, in a group, or virtually.
- ☐ Describe the clinical course including any interruption in or discontinuation of treatment.

- ☐ Disclose if the patient(s) received any type of simultaneous clinical service that could not be controlled and whose influence may have affected results.

Interveners

- ☐ Describe the type of professional(s) who provided treatment, the number of therapists involved in care, and the type and length of training that the therapist(s) received to administer intervention.
- ☐ If more than one therapist provided care, describe the procedures to ensure that all interveners provided intervention uniformly.

Data Collection

- ☐ Describe how, when, and by whom each set of data was collected.
- ☐ Disclose if the intervener also collected data.
- ☐ If multiple data collectors were used, detail how data collectors were trained to collect data uniformly and whether interrater reliability was established among data collectors.

Data Analysis

- ☐ Describe and cite all descriptive, statistical, and qualitative data analysis methods used to compare baseline and postintervention measures.
- ☐ Indicate at what statistical level probability was set.
- ☐ Describe and cite all qualitative data analysis methods used to understand patient satisfaction and perceptions of intervention.
- ☐ Name and cite all software programs used in data analysis.

Results

- ☐ Detail the findings of baseline, postintervention, and follow-up measures.
- ☐ Document the patient's perception of intervention on self-report measures and qualitative interviews.
- ☐ Supplement quantitative and qualitative data with information about gains the patient made in postintervention functional community participation.
- ☐ Organize the Results section in accordance with the order of case questions outlined in the purpose statement. Findings should be reported for each case question.
- ☐ When statistical analysis has been performed to compare baseline and postintervention measures, the statistical test results, *p* values, and confidence intervals should be reported.
- ☐ Support qualitative findings with quotations from the patient, family member, or caregiver.
- ☐ Report any adverse effects or unexpected findings.

Discussion

- ☐ Be careful not to overstate findings or generalize results beyond the patient(s).
- ☐ Organize the Discussion section according to the order of case questions provided in the purpose statement and addressed in the Results section.
- ☐ Attempt to explain all findings including unanticipated findings.

- ☐ Discuss adverse events as they relate to intervention safety and risk.
- ☐ Discuss how the case report or case series findings can inform future research needed to build consensus regarding best practice.

Limitations

- ☐ Discuss possible weaknesses in internal validity:
  - ☐ Possible lack of intervention fidelity if multiple interveners were used
  - ☐ Possible compromised anonymization if the intervener and data collector were the same therapist
  - ☐ Insufficient sample size power
  - ☐ Lack of control and randomization
  - ☐ Possible use of instruments with little or no established psychometric properties
- ☐ Discuss possible weaknesses in external validity:
  - ☐ Findings from one to three patients cannot be generalized beyond those patients
  - ☐ The use of patient incentives may have biased findings
- ☐ If follow-up points were not built into the case design, it is difficult to understand if patient gains resulting from intervention were maintained over time.

Future Directions

- ☐ Recommend the next steps that should follow after the case report or case series is completed. This may involve the recommendation of future research study designs that address the above-noted possible limitations.

Implications for Practice

- ☐ Indicate how findings can be used in practice decisions for the patient(s) in the case.
- ☐ Indicate how the present case findings can help to generate clinical questions that must be answered to develop best practice guidelines.
- ☐ Indicate how findings can be used to design future research studies with more rigorous designs.

Conclusions

- ☐ Summarize the major study findings and describe how these findings have potential to inform future research that can build consensus for best practice.

Examples of Well-Written Case Reports

Allan, L. G. (2025). A multisensory, interdisciplinary approach to visual neglect for enhancement of visual attention following basal ganglia hemorrhage: A case report. *Open Journal of Occupational Therapy, 13*(1), 1–17. https://doi.org/10.15453/2168-6408.2278

Gerhardt, N. M., Armstrong, J. P., Serruya, M. D., & Mulcahey, M. (2024). Outcomes of the NuroSleeve and occupational therapy on upper limb function of an individual with chronic hemiparesis following a stroke: A case report. *Open Journal of Occupational Therapy, 12*(1), 1–8. https://doi.org/10.15453/2168-6408.2166

Gutman, S. A., Raphael-Greenfield, E. I., Kerr, L., Siedlitz, E., & Wang, C. (2014). Using motor-based role-play to enhance social skills in a nonverbal adolescent with high functioning autism: A case report. *Occupational Therapy in Mental Health, 30*, 12–25. doi:10.1080/01642 12X.2014.878235

References

American Psychological Association. (2020). *Publication manual of the American Psychological Association* (6th ed.). Author.

Gagnier, J. J., Kienle, G., Altman, D. G., Moher, D., Sox, H., & Riley, D., for the CARE Group. (2013). The CARE Guidelines: Consensus-based clinical case reporting guideline development. *Global Advances in Health and Medicine*, *2*(5), 38–43. https://doi.org/10.7453/gahmj.2013.008

Mosey, A. C. (1996). *Applied scientific inquiry in the health professions: An epistemological orientation* (2nd ed.). American Occupational Therapy Association.

Riley, D. S., Barber, M. S., Kienle, G. S., Aronson, J. K., von Schoen-Angerer, T., Tugwell, P., Kiene, H., Helfand, M., Altman, D. G., Sox, H., & Werthmann, P. G. (2017). CARE guidelines for case reports: Explanation and elaboration document. *Journal of Clinical Epidemiology*, *89*, 218–235. https://doi.org/10.1016/j.jclinepi.2017.04.026

CHAPTER 9

Manuscript Structure and Content for Program Evaluations

Program evaluation manuscripts report the outcomes of a short program that was delivered to a specific group of patients (or clients) to meet a particular health care need. Program evaluations are not research studies, and they do not involve the rigor of intervention effectiveness studies. Because program evaluations are not research studies and can be completed in a much shorter length of time than intervention effectiveness studies, they make good capstone projects.

Most program evaluations provide intervention or health care education to one group of patients (or clients) in a single setting who share the same diagnosis, condition, or health care need. Outcome measures are collected at baseline (before the program begins) and at program end. Examples of program evaluations include (a) a literacy program for 1st graders in a low socioeconomic school district, who are reading below grade level; (b) a community participation program for refugee survivors of war who require assistance to resettle and become participating community members; and (c) a body image group for patients with burns who are experiencing body image dysmorphia.

Program evaluations are often the first step of trialing a novel intervention for a small group of patients (or clients) in everyday practice and do not involve the rigors of research design such as the use of comparison or control groups, random assignment to groups, participant sampling methods, anonymization of interveners and data collectors to participant groups, and institutional review board approval. Authors should, however, seek participant written consent to use their data in the author's capstone project.

Although program evaluations do not require the rigors of a research study, we recommend that authors, at a minimum, prepare a written protocol documenting each session's objective and content, length of sessions and number of sessions per week, and overall length of program. The following guidelines will help authors prepare a manuscript for program evaluations for capstone projects. Using the following headings and addressing the content that belongs in each will help authors ensure that they have included all critical information.

DOI: 10.4324/9781003734550-9

Program evaluation manuscripts should be approximately 5,000 words in length and 20 to 25 double-spaced, typed pages. The written protocol for the program evaluation can be placed in an appendix and is not counted as part of the 5,000-word length.

Manuscript Headings and Formatting for Program Evaluations

The following heading levels and formatting are based on American Psychological Association 7th edition (2020) guidelines.

Title

Begin the manuscript with a title on a separate title page. The title should be centered and typed in uppercase and lowercase letters.

Abstract

The Abstract should be placed on the page directly following the title page. The word *Abstract* should be capitalized, centered, and bolded.

Introduction

The Introduction begins on the page directly following the abstract. The heading *Introduction* is not typed in the manuscript because the beginning of the manuscript text alerts the reader that the Introduction has begun.

Literature Review

In a capstone project manuscript, the Literature Review follows the Introduction. The heading is bolded, capitalized, and flush left.

Description of the Program

In a capstone project manuscript, the Description of the Program follows the Literature Review. The heading is bolded, capitalized, and flush left.

Method

The Method section is positioned directly after the Introduction. The heading *Method* is centered, capitalized, and bolded.

Program Evaluation Design

Program Evaluation Design is the first subheading in the Method section. It is bolded, capitalized, and flush left.

Participants

Participants is the second subheading in the Method section. It is bolded, capitalized, and flush left.

Instruments (or Outcome Measures)

Instruments, or Outcome Measures, is the third subheading in the Method section. It is bolded, capitalized, and flush left.

Program Description

Program Description is the fourth subheading of the Method section. It is flush left, bolded, and capitalized.

Program Facilitators

Program Facilitators is the fifth heading of the Method section. It is flush left, bolded, and capitalized.

Data Collection

Data Collection is the sixth heading in the Method section. It is bolded, capitalized, and flush left.

Data Analysis

Data Analysis is the final heading in the Method section. It is bolded, capitalized, and flush left.

Results

The Results section directly follows Data Analysis and begins a new section of the paper. The heading *Results* is bolded, capitalized, and centered.

Discussion

The Discussion section directly follows the Results and begins a new section of the paper. The heading *Discussion* is bolded, capitalized, and centered.

Limitations

The Limitations subsection is part of the Discussion section but should be highlighted for the reader by a separate subheading within the Discussion section. The subheading *Limitations* is bolded, capitalized, and flush left.

Future Directions

The Future Directions subsection directly follows the Limitations subsection. This section is also part of the Discussion section and should be highlighted for the reader by a separate subheading label. The subheading *Future Directions* is bolded, capitalized, and flush left.

Implications for Practice

Implications for Practice is a subsection of the Discussion section and follows the Future Direction section. The subheading *Implications for Practice* is bolded, capitalized, and flush left.

Conclusion

The Conclusion is the final subsection of the Discussion and follows Implications for Practice. The heading is bolded, capitalized, and flush left.

References

References begin on a separate page following the Conclusion. The heading is centered, capitalized, and bolded.

Tables

Tables should be provided after the end of the references and begin on a separate page. Each table should be presented on its own page. Tables are named and presented in accordance with the order in which they are mentioned in the text. The title of the Table is inserted beneath the Table heading:

Table 1 [bolded, capitalized, and flush left]
Participant Demographics [italicized, capitalized, and flush left]

Figures

Figures should be provided after the end of the tables and begin on a separate page. Each figure should be presented on its own page. Figures are named and presented in accordance with the order in which they are mentioned in the text. The title of the Figure is inserted beneath the Figure heading:

Figure 1 [bolded, capitalized, and flush left]
Examples of Participant Quotes [italicized, capitalized, and flush left]

Manuscript Heading Content for Program Evaluations

There should be no repetition of content in the manuscript. The sections and subsections that follow next should not contain overlap and will not if written as suggested.

Title

The title of a program evaluation should contain four essential elements to assist readers to clearly understand the program and population addressed.

- Program name (i.e., the intervention). It is often good practice to include the length of the program (e.g., 10-week caregiver educational program).
- Participants
- Outcome measures (i.e., what is intended to be gained as a result of participation in the program?)
- The words "Program Evaluation" should appear in the title to indicate the design.

Examples of good program evaluation titles include the following:

- Assessing a 7-week Caregiver Education Program for Caregivers of Adults with Frontotemporal Dementia: A Program Evaluation
- Assessing a 3-month Body Image Program for Adolescents with Burn Injuries and Body Dysmorphia: A Program Evaluation
- A 12-week Program to Help Young Adults with Substance Use Histories to Replace Use Behaviors with Functional and Meaningful Occupations: A Program Evaluation

Abbreviations in the title should be avoided unless commonly used and understood in the health care community.

Writing Exercises: Titles

- Practice writing a title for your program evaluation manuscript using the above guidelines and examples.
- Identify the program, participants, and desired outcome and combine these into one title. Include the words "Program Evaluation" to indicate the design.
- Ask a peer who does not know much about your project to read your title and tell you what they think your paper is about. If the reader is correct, you have likely written an adequate title. If they are not correct or are confused, you may need to revise your title using the above directions.

Abstract

The abstract of a program evaluation manuscript is best organized using the following subheadings: (a) objectives, (b) method, (c) results, and (d) conclusions. Addressing the specific content of each subheading, as recommended next, will ensure that you provide readers with critical information needed to understand the program's objective, participants, outcome measures, and results. An abstract for a program evaluation should be approximately 150–200 words.

- Objectives: In one to two sentences, authors should describe the intended purpose of the program. The program length should be included (e.g., 10-week community participation program).
- Method: In one to two sentences, authors should provide information about participants (e.g., clinical diagnosis or condition, number participating, how participants were obtained), program evaluation design (e.g., one group pre- and post-program measures), and outcome measures (e.g., baseline and post-program Likert scale surveys).
- Results: In one to two sentences, authors should report the primary findings. If basic statistical analysis was used, authors should report statistical test results, *p* values, and confidence intervals when appropriate.

- Conclusions: In one to two sentences, authors should (a) describe the implications of their findings for the participants and (b) address how the findings can be used to generate next steps for continued development and assessment of the program.

Abstract example:

Objective: The purpose of this program evaluation was to assess a 12-week after-school program that assisted 7 high school students in a low socioeconomic school district to remain in school until the academic year end, enhance academic skills, and begin to plan post-secondary goals.

Method: Seven high school students who were in danger of dropping out of school were selected to participate in the program by the school guidance counselor. Outcome measures included number of days of school attendance, academic grades, completion of the school year, and the establishment of 3 feasible post-secondary goals—all measured pre- and post-program.

Results: Five students completed the program and the school year. The average school attendance for the 5 students increased from 3 days per week to 5. Grade point average increased from C- to B. All 5 students established 3 feasible post-secondary goals including entering vocational training programs and community college.

Conclusion: Findings suggest that the 12-week after-school program was able to help 5 students avert school dropout and successfully complete the school year. A follow-up program will assist the students in the steps needed to explore, apply to, and enter vocational training and community college programs.

Writing Exercises: Abstract [approximately 150–200 words]

- The abstract is the last section that should be written after all other manuscript sections are completed.
- Practice writing an abstract for your manuscript using the provided guidelines.
- Objectives: Go to the purpose statement of your manuscript and identify the purpose of the program evaluation. Modify this sentences(s) so that it is not taken verbatim from the manuscript text.
- Method: Go to your Methods section of your manuscript and identify information regarding the following: participants (e.g., diagnosis or condition, number, how participants were obtained), program evaluation design, and data collection procedures. Revise these sentences so that they are not written verbatim and can be shortened and combined into one to two sentences.
- Results: Select the primary findings from your Results section. You will likely not be able to report all of your findings in the abstract. Select approximately two primary results that are most salient to your manuscript. Try to rewrite these sentences so that they are shortened into one to two sentences. If basic statistical analysis was used, each result should be accompanied by the statistical test result, exact p value, and confidence interval when appropriate.

- Conclusions: Go to your Discussion section and select one to two primary points regarding the implications of your findings for your participants and the program. Rewrite these sentences so that they are shortened into one to two sentences.
- Ask a peer who is not familiar with your project to read your abstract and let you know if it is clear, and if not, what can be made clearer. Make revisions as needed and repeat the process of obtaining feedback and making revisions.

Introduction [no heading needed]

The Introduction of a program evaluation manuscript is approximately four to five double-spaced, typed pages. The Introduction includes the background, need for the program, literature review, description of the program, purpose statement, and project questions. The background describes the problem or situation that a clinical population is experiencing and for which the program has been designed as a possible intervention. The background often begins with statistics regarding prevalence or incidence of the clinical condition or situation.

The need for the program answers the questions, "Why is this program needed for this particular clinical population? How will the program assist the patients or clients who are participating?"

Writing Exercises: Introduction

Background [approximately 2–3 paragraphs]

- Practice writing the Introduction section of your manuscript. Begin by describing the background of the problem as it relates to the clinical population addressed. Most backgrounds begin with information about prevalence or incidence rate of the addressed clinical condition.
- Describe the current problem with regard to the clinical population's daily life function, community participation, or some other important aspect of their life situation. How have these factors impacted the addressed clinical population?
- Then describe how this problem has impacted the larger society and the profession.

Need for the Program [commonly 2 paragraphs]

- The need for the program answers the questions, "Why is this program needed now to help the addressed clinical population?" "How will the program assist the patients or clients who are participating to enhance their desired daily life activities and community participation?"
- For a program evaluation, the need for the program will often address the assessment of (a) a novel intervention program for a specific clinical population that has not been assessed or (b) an existing intervention program that was designed for one clinical population and that needs to be assessed with a different clinical population.

Once you have drafted the background and need statement, ask a peer to read your work and describe the background and need for your study. If the reader could not adequately describe the background and need as you intended, identify what they missed and rewrite those components.

Once you have revised the background and need statement, repeat this last step with another peer who is unfamiliar with your study.

Literature Review

The Literature Review is approximately two to three double-spaced, typed pages and provides a synthesis of all published studies that report intervention methods intended to address the identified problem or situation. Authors should describe the results of previous studies documenting intervention attempts to aid the clinical condition or situation. Authors should also identify existing knowledge gaps regarding intervention for the clinical condition or situation and clearly state how the present program evaluation will generate information needed to aid the participants in the present program. Because program evaluations are not research studies and do not possess the rigor of randomization, control/comparison, and anonymization, authors can only state that the results of program evaluation can provide information needed to help the participants in the present program.

The 7-year rule applies to program evaluations—articles reviewed in all sections of the Introduction should have been published within the last 7 years; however, classic studies or theoretical papers that were published more than 7 years ago are the exception to this rule. Because many health care professions are in their early evolution in the building of evidence, intervention studies published within the last 7 years may be lacking or insufficient to make best practice decisions. When this is the case, authors should clearly describe this deficiency in the Literature Review.

Writing Exercises: Literature Review [commonly 2–3 double-spaced, typed pages]

- See Chapter 3 for more details about writing different types of literature reviews.
- Go to the literature and complete a database search on your topic using keywords. Identify all studies within a specified time period that directly relate to your program evaluation and targeted population.
- The literature review should synthesize the current published information regarding intervention attempts with your targeted population so that readers can gain an understanding of what research has been completed to date and what may be lacking.
- Generally, a synthesis means that you will summarize the existing literature using larger categories such as research design, specific population, sample size,

findings, and limitations. It may be helpful for you to make a chart to organize this data so that you can present it in narrative form.
- When only a handful (≤5) of intervention studies exist, authors may present more specific information about each of these studies instead of synthesizing them as a group.
- Literature reviews should end with a paragraph about what information is missing from the existing literature and how your program evaluation intends to fill this gap in the profession's knowledge base.
- Ask a peer, ideally a health care professional who is familiar with your topic, to read your literature review and provide feedback about its exhaustiveness and clarity.
- Make revisions based on the provided feedback. Repeat the process of seeking feedback and making revisions.

Description of the Program

Following the Literature Review, authors should provide a short description of the intervention program, the theoretical bases that were used to develop the program, and a brief narrative describing how the intervention program is intended to be used with the identified population (e.g., general program content, delivery methods, appropriate settings). Information about overall program length, number of sessions per week, and length of each session—or what is typically referred to as dosage and duration—will be described in the Method section.

Writing Exercises: Description of the Program [approximately 1–3 paragraphs]

- When an intervention program is novel and has been developed for a specific population, authors should provide a description of the intervention, its theoretical base, and proposed delivery methods.
- Authors should state that they developed this novel intervention to meet a treatment need that was lacking for a specific clinical population in a particular setting.
- Describe and cite the theoretical bases that were used to develop the intervention.
- Describe the intervention as it is intended to be used with the specific clinical population identified. The description should involve program content, delivery methods (e.g., one-to-one therapy, group therapy, video instruction, virtual reality methods), and settings in which the program is intended to be delivered.
- Do not describe details such as overall length of intervention, number of sessions per week, and length of each session, or what is typically referred to as dosage and duration. These details will be placed in the Method section.

- Ask a peer, ideally a health care professional, to read your intervention description and describe it back to you offering such details as the population for which the intervention program was intended, the content of the program, settings in which the program was meant to be delivered, and delivery methods. If the reader provided these details accurately, you have likely written a good description of your program. If the reader missed or confused details, ask them to identify what was unclear and use this feedback to revise your program description.
- Once a second draft has been written, repeat the process of seeking feedback and making revisions with another peer.

Final Paragraph Before Method [no heading needed]

The purpose statement is the final paragraph of the Introduction and is inserted after the Description of the Program. Here, authors should state the purpose of the program evaluation and provide clear and precise questions. Questions for a program evaluation manuscript should contain the targeted population, program, and outcome measures. Questions commonly pertain to such items as effect, client satisfaction and perceptions, and tolerance. Examples of good program evaluation questions include the following:

- Can a 12-week after school mentoring program for adolescents in a low socioeconomic school district and who are at risk for school failure, help students to increase their school attendance, complete the academic year, enhance grade point average, and establish three feasible postsecondary education/employment goals?
- What do students perceive as the most helpful components of the program and why? What were the least helpful and how could these be enhanced?
- What do students identify as missing components of the program that could be added?
- What do students identify as facilitating their completion of the program?
- What do students identify as barriers to their completion of the program and how can these barriers be ameliorated?

Writing Exercises: Purpose Statement

- Practice writing a purpose statement for your program evaluation manuscript. Begin with "The purpose of this program evaluation was to ..." and complete the sentence with the primary objective of your project.
- Example: "The purpose of the present program evaluation was to assess the parent perceptions of a program designed to help parents interact with their children with ASD in daily activities and games that could enhance communication skills."
- Remember that all program evaluation manuscripts are written in the past tense.

Writing Exercises: Program Evaluation Questions

- Practice writing questions for your program evaluation using the guidelines above.
- Make sure to include the clinical population, program intervention, and outcome measures.
- Ask a peer to read your program evaluation questions and then explain what you are seeking through your project. If the reader is accurate, you have likely written good research questions. If they are not accurate, you may want to revise your questions based on the labeling strategies outlined above.

Definitions

All new and unfamiliar terms that are presented in the Introduction (and throughout the text) should be defined when the term first appears in the manuscript. Common mistakes include failing to define terms, unclearly defining terms, presenting terms in one section and defining them in another, and changing the definition of a term in a paper.

Good definitions contain three elements (Mosey, 1996):

1. Label
2. Superordinate concept
3. Distinguishing characteristics

The label is the term used to describe a specific concept. The label chosen should be used consistently throughout the paper and should not change.

The superordinate concept is the larger umbrella term or category under which the term falls.

Distinguishing characteristics are the concepts that differentiate the term from similar concepts.

Examples of good definitions include the following:

- Repetitive strain disorders [label] are overuse syndromes [superordinate concept] in which the soft tissues of a joint become inflamed as a result of repeated engagement in activities that require continued movement [distinguishing concepts].
- Cognitive problem-solving strategies [label] are executive functions mediated by the frontal lobe [superordinate concept] that require the ability to identify a problem, plan a strategy, execute the strategy, evaluate the strategy's effect, and modify the strategy as needed [distinguishing characteristics].
- Food refusal [label] is the rejection of specific food types [superordinate concept] based on tastes, textures, consistencies, scents, and appearances that are aversive to the child [distinguishing concepts].

Writing Exercises: Definitions

- Make sure that all new and unfamiliar terms for readers are defined in your manuscript when they first appear. If you are unsure about which terms may be new or unfamiliar to readers, ask a peer to read your work and identify such terms.
- Practice writing good definitions using the guidelines above and ensuring that you have a label, superordinate category, and distinguishing characteristics for all new and unfamiliar terms.
- To practice, define the term *occupational therapy*.
- Occupational therapy [label] is a health care profession [superordinate category] that assists people to restore or newly gain participation in desired daily life activities in home and community settings through skilled services, remediation, adaptation, and compensation [distinguishing characteristics].
- After writing several definitions, ask a peer to read them and let you know if they are clear. If they are not clear, ask the reader why or what part of the definition is unclear.
- Then revise the definitions with that feedback. Continue to use labels, superordinate categories, and distinguishing characteristics to structure your revised definitions. Repeat the process of seeking feedback and making revisions.

Quotations

Quotations should not be used in health science scholarly writing with the exception of the following:

- Quoting historical or legal documents
- Quoting a technical definition that has been accepted by the scientific community and whose meaning may significantly change if the exact wording is altered
- Quoting a participant's response in a qualitative study

With the exception of the above instances, quotations should not be used. Instead, authors should paraphrase content and cite the source.

Method

Providing clear, detailed, and precise methods is critical for practitioners to (a) assess the congruency between a program evaluation's objectives and procedures; (b) understand whether an intervention can be applied to their own clients and clinical setting; and (c) replicate the program as intended with similar or different clinical populations. The use of the following subheadings in the Method section, and the content belonging in each subheading, will help you to provide critical information that practitioners need to accomplish the above.

Program Evaluation Design

The Method section of program evaluation manuscripts should begin with a subheading labeled *Program Evaluation Design*. Most program evaluation designs are one-group pretest/posttest designs that occur in the real life of a clinical setting. One group of clients participates in a program and pre-program and post-program measures are collected. When program evaluations are carried out as part of a capstone project, authors should obtain written consent from participants (or their parents or guardians) to collect and disseminate their aggregate data through the capstone written paper and presentation. Authors should state that written informed consent was obtained. Since capstone program evaluations are not research studies, they do not require institutional review board approval.

Writing Exercises: Program Evaluation Design [approximately 1 paragraph]

- Write the Program Evaluation Design section of your Methods making sure to
  - Describe the design—usually a one-group pretest/posttest design.
  - State that informed consent was attained from adult participants or assent from child participants (or both when appropriate).
- Ask a peer to read your Program Evaluation Design section and let you know if it is clear and contains all needed information. Make revisions as needed.

Participants

Most program evaluations commonly take place in real-life clinical settings with participants who are already clients receiving services within the setting. In some settings a group of clients may already be assembled, whereas in other settings participants may need to be recruited. The Participants section should detail the recruitment strategy and indicate the setting from which participants came. If there are any inclusion/exclusion criteria that detail who can and cannot participate in the program, these should also be explicitly stated for the reader. If participation in the program was open to any client already receiving services in a specific setting, this should also be made clear for readers. Authors should additionally disclose who recruited and selected participants and their relationship to participants. The setting from which clients were selected should be described with regard to facility type and size, provided services, approximate length of admission or residency, and geographical region.

Note that participant demographics, participant flow, and final sample size are part of the results and should be documented in the Results section rather than the Method section.

Writing Exercises: Participants [approximately 1–2 paragraphs]

- Write the Participants section of your Methods making sure to
  - Describe how participants were recruited and selected.
  - Detail any inclusion/exclusion criteria.
  - State who completed participant recruitment and selection and their relationship to participants.
  - If the program was open to any client already receiving services in a specific setting, this should be stated.
  - Describe the setting from which participants were recruited with regard to facility type and size, provided services, approximate length of admission or residency, and geographical region.
- Ask a peer to read your Participants section and describe who your targeted participant group was, recruitment and selection methods, the setting from which participants were recruited, and any inclusion/exclusion criteria.
- If your reader could easily identify these, you have likely written a good Participants section. If they could not, revise your Participants section using the above guidelines. Repeat the process of obtaining feedback and making revisions.

Instruments

The Instruments, or Outcome Measures, section describes the instruments that were used to measure outcomes. Instruments should be described in detail so that readers can evaluate whether a selected instrument was appropriate to measure a specific outcome. Instruments should be described with regard to purpose, intended population, type of data collected (e.g., self-report, performance-based observer rating, Likert scale, open-ended questions, or total score yielding ratio data), and administration length. The instrument's psychometric properties relating to reliability and validity should be provided in numeric values with statistical test results, *p* values, and confidence intervals indicated. Authors should not singularly state that an instrument's reliability or validity is *high*; instead, readers should be provided with the numeric values of statistical tests so that they can evaluate the instrument themselves. Both the instrument and its psychometric properties should be cited. If psychometric properties for an instrument have not been established, or if an instrument has been newly developed for the present program evaluation, authors should clearly state this information. Similarly, if authors have developed an instrument for the present program evaluation, they should describe the development process and indicate whether an attempt was made to establish face or content validity through the evaluation of an expert panel. For a capstone project, the newly developed instrument can be provided in a figure or appendix.

Outcome measures that are assessed using frequency counts or participant qualitative responses are appropriate for program evaluations. Such outcome measures should be described but do not possess psychometric properties that must be detailed.

Writing Exercises: Instruments [approximately 1–3 paragraphs depending on how many instruments/outcome measures were used]

- Write the Instruments section of your Methods making sure to
  - Describe all instruments used to measure study outcomes with regard to
    - Intended purpose
    - Population for which the instrument was designed and assessed
    - Type of data collected
    - Length of administration
  - Provide the citation(s) for all instruments
  - Report the reliability and validity for all instruments. Provide numeric values for statistical test results along with exact *p* values and confidence intervals. Provide citations for reliability and validity data.
  - If an instrument was developed for the present program evaluation, this should be stated, and authors should describe the instrument development process. The instrument can be provided in a figure or appendix.
  - Outcome measures that are assessed using frequency counts or participant qualitative responses should also be described for readers.
- Ask a peer who understands research methods to read your Instruments section and let you know if they understand each instrument's purpose, intended population, type of data that can be collected, administration length, and reliability and validity. If the reader cannot, ask what is unclear and use that feedback to revise your work.

Program Description

Authors should describe the program with regard to the number and length of sessions (dose); length of the entire program (duration); content of each session; whether sessions were delivered individually, in a group, or both; and whether and how the program was tailored for specific clients. Authors should also disclose whether clients received any type of simultaneous clinical service that could have influenced results.

Writing Exercises: Program Description [approximately 1–3 paragraphs]

- Write a first draft of your Program Description section making sure to describe the program with regard to
  - Number and length of sessions (dose)
  - Length of the entire program (duration)
  - Content of each session

- Whether sessions were delivered individually, in a group, or both
- Disclose whether clients received any type of simultaneous clinical service that could have influenced results.

- Once you have a first draft of your Program Description section, ask a peer to read it and describe all elements of the program to you. If the reader can accurately do so, you have likely written a thorough Program Description section.
- If the reader identifies anything that is unclear about the description of the program, use this information to make revisions and repeat the process of seeking feedback and making revisions with another peer.

Program Facilitators

Key information should be provided about the professionals who administered the program. Authors should report who facilitated the program, type of professional(s), number of professionals involved in program delivery, professionals' experience level, and type of training received to facilitate the program.

Writing Exercises: Program Facilitators [approximately 1 paragraph]

- Write a first draft of your Program Facilitator section making sure to include
  - Who facilitated the program
  - Type of professional(s)
  - Number of professionals involved in program delivery
  - Professionals' experience level
  - Type of training received to facilitate the program
- Once you have a first draft of your Program Facilitators section, ask a peer to read it and describe all information about who the facilitators were. If the reader can accurately do so, you have likely written a thorough Program Facilitators section.
- Ask the reader to identify if there is anything that is unclear about the descriptions of the facilitators and use this information to make revisions. Repeat the process of seeking feedback and making revisions with another peer.

Data Collection

The Data Collection subsection should detail how, when, and by whom each set of data in the study was collected. In a program evaluation for a capstone project, it is common for the author to both facilitate the program and collect data; however, such overlap of roles should be clearly stated because this condition may introduce bias and influence results. If more than one data collector was used, authors should detail whether and how data collectors were trained to collect data uniformly.

Writing Exercises: Data Collection [approximately 2–3 paragraphs]

- Write a first draft of your Data Collection section making sure to
  - Report the data collection schedule describing how, when, and by whom each set of data was collected.
  - Disclose whether the program facilitator also collected data. This situation is common in program evaluations but should be disclosed because of the possible bias that may influence findings.
  - If more than one data collector was used, describe how data collectors were trained to collect data uniformly.
- Ask a peer to read your Data Collection section and let you know if it is clear and contains all needed information. Ask the reader to identify what is missing or confusing. Use this feedback to make revisions.

Data Analysis

All descriptive, statistical, and qualitative data analysis methods used to compare baseline and post-program measures, and analyze the participants' perceptions of the program, should be described and cited. The names and citations of all analytic software programs should also be provided, and the level at which statistical significance was set for quantitative tests should be reported.

Writing Exercises: Data Analysis [approximately 2–3 paragraphs]

- Write the Data Analysis section of your Methods making sure to
  - Describe and cite all descriptive, statistical, and qualitative data analysis methods used to compare baseline and post-program measures.
  - Indicate at what statistical level probability was set.
  - Describe and cite all qualitative data analysis methods used to understand participant satisfaction with and perceptions of the program.
  - Name and cite all software programs used in data analysis.
- Ask a peer to read your Data Analysis section and let you know if it is clear and contains all needed information. Ask the reader to identify what is missing or confusing. Use this feedback to make revisions.

The Method section should be approximately five double-spaced, typed pages in length.

Results

The Results section should begin with a description of participant flow including the number of participants enrolled in the program, the number who withdrew from the program, and the number who completed the program. Information about why participants withdrew from program participation should be reported if known.

Authors should report participant demographics with regard to age, gender, race, ethnicity, education level, socioeconomic level, and topic-specific characteristics such as functional level and independent living status. When demographics are reported, absolute numbers should be provided. If percentages are used, the absolute numbers from which the percentages were derived should be provided. If any of the above-noted demographics were not collected, authors should disclose this.

After reporting participant flow and demographics, the Results section should be organized in accordance with the order of program evaluation questions outlined in the purpose statement. Findings should be reported for each program evaluation question. Most quantitative outcome measures in a program evaluation will be analyzed and reported using descriptive statistics (e.g., mean, median, mode, range, standard deviation). If more advanced statistics were used to measure the difference between pre- and post-program test scores, the statistical test value, p value, and confidence interval should be provided.

Make sure to report findings without interpreting them. Interpretation of findings will be made in the Discussion section.

When reporting qualitative data addressing such items as participant satisfaction and perceptions of program delivery, authors should collate data according to program evaluation questions and provide participant quotes to support collective findings.

If any adverse effects or unexpected findings occurred during program delivery, these should be reported.

See Chapter 10, Reporting Statistical Data in Text and Tables, to understand how to correctly report statistical tests and symbols in the Results section.

The Results section should be between three and four double-spaced pages in length.

Writing Exercises: Results [approximately 3–4 double spaced, typed pages]

- Use the checklist at the end of this chapter to make an outline of your Results section.
- Then order your program evaluation questions in accordance with the order outlined in the purpose statement. Beneath each question, insert the primary points that you want to include. Report findings for each program evaluation question.
- Using your outline, write the Results section making sure to
  - Begin with information about participant flow and demographics.
  - For each quantitative outcome measure calculated with advanced statistics, report the statistical test value, p value, and confidence interval.
  - Report all findings without interpreting them. Interpretation will be made in the Discussion section.
  - Report descriptive statistical results using absolute numbers. If percentages are used, also report the absolute numbers from which the percentages were derived.

- When reporting qualitative data addressing such items as participant satisfaction and perceptions of program delivery, collate data according to program evaluation questions. Provide participant quotes to support qualitative findings.
- Report unanticipated and adverse events that occurred as a result of program delivery.

- Finally, ask a peer to read your Results section and describe it back to you, indicating what is clear and what needs greater clarification. Make revisions based on that feedback. Repeat the process of seeking feedback and making revisions with another peer.

Discussion

The Discussion section in a program evaluation allows authors to interpret the findings reported in the Results section as they relate to the program participants. It is important that authors do not overstate their findings about the program's effect because program evaluations lack the rigor of control/comparison, randomization, larger sample sizes, and anonymization procedures. In a program evaluation, authors can only state that the program appeared to have an effect on the participants. While generalization of findings cannot be made, authors can suggest that the program shows promise and warrants future study with larger sample sizes and more rigorous study methods. The Discussion section should be organized according to the order of program evaluation questions provided in the purpose statement and addressed in the Results section. Authors should attempt to answer each program evaluation question based on findings presented in the Results section. Unanticipated findings should be explained, and the occurrence of adverse events should be examined with regard to program risk and safety. Authors should discuss how the program evaluation findings can inform future research needed to build consensus regarding best practice.

Writing Exercises: Discussion [approximately 4–5 doubled-spaced, typed pages]

- Use the checklist at the end of this chapter to make an outline of your Discussion section.
- Make sure to address the following:
  - Organize your Discussion section in accordance with the order of program evaluation questions in your purpose statement and Results section. Interpret the findings for each program evaluation question.
  - Explain and interpret all findings without repeating the results. Why might each finding have occurred? Make sure that each program evaluation question is answered.

- Explain all unanticipated findings and the occurrence of adverse events as they relate to program risk and safety.
- In a program evaluation, authors can only state that the program appeared to have effect with the participants. It is important not to overstate findings.
- Although generalization of the findings from program evaluations cannot be made to the larger population, authors can suggest that the program shows promise and warrants future study with larger sample sizes and more rigorous study methods.
- Suggest how the program evaluation findings can inform future research needed to build consensus regarding best practice.

- Ask a peer to read your Discussion section and let you know if it is clear and contains all needed information. Ask the reader to identify what is missing or confusing. Use this feedback to make revisions. Repeat the process of seeking feedback and making revisions with another peer until the Discussion is complete.

Limitations

Program evaluations have inherent weaknesses in internal and external validity that should be documented in the Limitations section.

Weaknesses in internal validity (i.e., the degree to which researchers can be confident that the changes in outcome measures were a result of the intervention) include the following:

- The results may have been biased if more than one program facilitator was used and did not deliver the program uniformly and as intended (i.e., possible lack of intervention fidelity).
- The results may have been biased if the program facilitator also collected data.
- The results may have been biased by a small participant size.
- The results may have been biased by a lack of control and randomization procedures.
- The results may have been biased by the use of instruments with little or no established psychometric properties.

Weaknesses in external validity (i.e., the degree to which researchers can be confident that the participants represent the larger population) include the following:

- The use of incentives to participate in the program may have changed the participants' experience of program delivery.
- A small participant group cannot be assumed to represent the larger population.

One further limitation may involve the lack of follow-up points to determine if the participant gains made at program end were maintained over time.

Writing Exercises: Limitations [approximately 1 paragraph]

- Use the checklist at the end of this chapter to make an outline of your Limitations section.
- Determine if any of the following weaknesses apply to your program evaluation and should be documented in the Limitations section:
  - Results may have been biased if multiple facilitators participated in program delivery and varied in the uniformity of program delivery.
  - Potential bias may have impacted the results if the program facilitator also collected data.
  - Lack of control and randomization may have biased results because the participants may not represent the larger population.
  - The possible use of instruments with little or no established psychometric properties may have biased results because it is not clear what such instruments truly measured.
  - Participant incentives may have biased results because such incentives may have changed the participants, making them different from the larger population.
  - Generalization to the larger population cannot be made from a small group of participants.
- If follow-up points were not used, it is difficult to understand if patient gains resulting from the program were maintained over time.
- Ask a peer to read your Discussion section and let you know if it is clear and contains all needed information. Ask the reader to identify what is missing or confusing. Use this feedback to make revisions.

Future Directions

Authors should suggest how future studies can address the present program evaluation's limitations and identify which questions regarding program delivery must still be answered. For example, is the program cost- and time-efficient? Can patients tolerate the program, and if not, how can it be improved? Although the program has been found to be effective with adults, can it be used with adolescents having the same clinical condition or situation? The Future Directions section is approximately one paragraph.

Writing Exercises: Future Directions [approximately 1–2 paragraphs]

- Use the checklist at the end of this chapter to make an outline of the main points in your Future Direction section.
- Write a first draft of the Future Direction section of your Discussion making sure to
  - Describe how future research can address the present program evaluation's limitations.

  - Identify program evaluation questions that remain unanswered and suggest directions for future studies.
- Ask a peer to read your Future Direction section and describe it back to you, indicating what is clear and what needs greater clarification. Make revisions based on that feedback.
- Write a second draft and repeat the process of obtaining feedback and making revisions if needed.

Implications for Practice

Implications for Practice can only relate to the participants in the program and their own clinical course over time, how findings from the program evaluation can be used to refine the program for future participants, and how findings can be used to design future research with more rigorous methodologies. This section is approximately one paragraph or 4–6 bullets.

The format for the Implications for Practice section is commonly presented as a narrative paragraph or bulleted list. The shortness of this section is a recognition that program evaluation findings have been derived from one sample that cannot be generalized to the larger population, and that further research must be conducted to add to the body of knowledge regarding the topic area.

Writing Exercises: Implications for Practice [approximately 1 paragraph or 4–6 bullets]

- Use the checklist at the end of this chapter to make an outline of the main points in your Implications for Practice section.
- Write a first draft of the Implications for Practice section of your Discussion making sure to relate the implications only to
  - The participants in the program and their own clinical course over time
  - How findings from the program evaluation can be used to refine the program for future participants
  - How findings can be used to design future research with more rigorous methodologies
- Ask a peer to read your Implications for Practice section and describe it back to you, indicating what is clear and what needs greater clarification. Also ask the reader to provide feedback regarding whether your implications for practice are overstated or inappropriately generalized to the larger population. Make revisions based on that feedback.
- If needed, write a second draft and repeat the process of obtaining feedback and making revisions.

Conclusion

In this final section of a program evaluation, authors should summarize the major findings and describe how these findings have potential to inform future program delivery with other participants and future research that can build consensus about practice decisions.

Writing Exercises: Conclusion [approximately 1–2 paragraphs]

- Use the checklist at the end of this chapter to make an outline of the main points in your Conclusion section.
- Write the Conclusion section making sure to
  - Summarize the study's primary findings as they relate to (a) the present participants, (b) how findings can be used to refine the program for future participants, and (c) how future research can be designed to assess the program using more rigorous methods.
  - Make sure not to overstate study findings or generalize them to the larger population.
- Ask a peer to read your Conclusion section and describe it back to you, indicating what is clear and what needs greater clarification. Make revisions based on that feedback.
- If needed, write a second draft and repeat the process of obtaining feedback and making revisions.

A concisely and well-written Discussion section should be approximately four to five double-spaced, typed pages in length.

After the Conclusion, the remaining manuscript sections in the order in which they should be presented are as follows:

- References
- Tables
- Figures

Checklist for Manuscript Structure and Content of Program Evaluations

Title

- ☐ Include the following elements: program name and length, participants, outcome measures, and the words *program evaluation*.

Abstract

- ☐ Objectives: In one to two sentences, describe the intended purpose of the program. The program length should be included (e.g., 10-week community participation program).

- ☐ Method: In one to two sentences, authors should provide information about participants (e.g., clinical diagnosis or condition, number participating, how participants were obtained), program evaluation design (e.g., one group pretest/posttest), and outcome measures (e.g., baseline and post-program Likert scale surveys).
- ☐ Results: In one to two sentences, authors should report the primary findings. If advanced statistical analysis was used authors should report statistical test results, *p* values, and confidence intervals when appropriate.
- ☐ Conclusions: In one to two sentences, authors should (a) describe the implications of their findings for the participants and (b) address how the findings can be used to generate next steps for continued development and assessment of the program.

Introduction [no heading needed]

- ☐ Begin by describing the background of the problem as it relates to the clinical population addressed. Most backgrounds begin with information about prevalence or incidence rate of the addressed clinical condition.
- ☐ Describe the current problem with regard to the clinical population's daily life function, community participation, or some other important aspect of their life situation. How have these factors impacted the addressed clinical population?
- ☐ Describe how this problem has impacted the larger society and the profession.
- ☐ Describe the need for the program. For a program evaluation, the need for the program will often address the assessment of (a) a novel intervention program for a specific clinical population that has not been assessed or (b) an existing intervention program that was designed for one clinical population and that needs to be assessed with a different clinical population.

Literature Review

- ☐ Synthesize the current published information regarding intervention attempts with your targeted population so that readers can gain an understanding of what research has been completed to date and what may be lacking.
- ☐ Literature reviews should end with a paragraph about what information is missing from the existing literature and how your program evaluation intends to fill this gap in the profession's knowledge base.

Description of the Program

- ☐ Authors should state that they developed this novel intervention program to meet a treatment need that was lacking for a specific clinical population in a particular setting.
- ☐ Describe and cite the theoretical bases that were used to develop the intervention.
- ☐ Describe the intervention program as it is intended to be used with the specific clinical population identified. The description should involve program content, delivery methods (e.g., one-to-one therapy, group therapy, video instruction, virtual reality methods), and settings in which the program is intended to be delivered.

Final Paragraph of Introduction [no heading is needed]

- ☐ Purpose statement: state the purpose of the program evaluation.
- ☐ Program evaluation questions: Questions for a program evaluation manuscript should contain the targeted population, program name, and outcome measures. Questions commonly pertain to such items as effect, client satisfaction and perceptions, and tolerance.

Method

Program Evaluation Design

- ☐ Describe the program evaluation design. Most program evaluation designs are one-group pretest/posttest designs that occur in the real life of a clinical setting.
- ☐ State that informed written consent was obtained from participants (or their parents or guardians) to collect and disseminate their aggregate data through the capstone written paper and presentation.

Participants

- ☐ Describe how participants were recruited and selected.
- ☐ Detail any inclusion/exclusion criteria.
- ☐ State who completed participant recruitment and selection.
- ☐ If the program was open to any client already receiving services in a specific setting, this should be stated.
- ☐ Describe the setting from which participants were recruited with regard to facility type and size, provided services, approximate length of admission or residency, and geographical region.

Instruments

- ☐ Describe all instruments used to measure study outcomes with regard to intended purpose, population for which the instrument was designed and assessed, type of data collected, and length of administration.
- ☐ Provide citation(s) for all instruments.
- ☐ Report the reliability and validity for all instruments. Provide numeric values for statistical test results along with exact p values and confidence intervals. Provide citations for reliability and validity data.
- ☐ If an instrument was developed for the present program evaluation, this should be stated and authors should describe the instrument development process. The instrument can be provided in a figure or appendix.
- ☐ Outcome measures that are assessed using frequency counts or participant qualitative responses should also be described for readers.

Program Description

- ☐ Describe the program with regard to the number and length of sessions (dose); length of the entire program (duration); content of each session; whether sessions were delivered individually, in a group, or both; and whether and how the program was tailored for specific clients.
- ☐ Disclose whether clients received any type of simultaneous clinical services that could have influenced results.

Program Facilitators

- ☐ Report who facilitated the program, type of professional(s), number of professionals involved in program delivery, professionals' experience level, and type of training received to facilitate the program.

Data Collection

- ☐ Report the data collection schedule describing how, when, and by whom each set of data was collected.
- ☐ Disclose whether the program facilitator also collected data. This situation is common in program evaluations but should be disclosed because of the possible bias that may influence findings.
- ☐ If more than one data collector was used, describe how data collectors were trained to collect data uniformly.

Data Analysis

- ☐ Describe and cite all descriptive, statistical, and qualitative data analysis methods used to compare baseline and post-program measures.
- ☐ Indicate at what statistical level probability was set.
- ☐ Describe and cite all qualitative data analysis methods used to understand participant satisfaction with and perceptions of the program.
- ☐ Name and cite all software programs used in data analysis.

Results

- ☐ Order your program evaluation questions in accordance with the order outlined in the purpose statement. Report findings for each program evaluation question.
- ☐ Begin with a description of participant flow including the number of participants enrolled in the program, the number who withdrew from the program, and the number included in the final analysis.
- ☐ Information about why participants withdrew from program participation should be reported if known.
- ☐ Authors should report participant demographics with regard to age, gender, race, ethnicity, education level, socioeconomic level, and topic-specific characteristics such as functional level and independent living status.
- ☐ For each advanced statistical tests used in analysis, report the statistical test value, *p* value, and confidence interval.
- ☐ Report all findings without interpreting them. Interpretation will be made in the Discussion section.
- ☐ Report descriptive quantitative results using absolute numbers. If percentages are used, also report the absolute numbers from which the percentages were derived.
- ☐ When reporting qualitative data addressing such items as participant satisfaction and perceptions of program delivery, collate data according to program evaluation questions. Provide participant quotes to support qualitative findings.
- ☐ Report unanticipated and adverse events that occurred as a result of program delivery.

Discussion

- ☐ Organize your Discussion section in accordance with the order of program evaluation questions in your purpose statement and Results section. Interpret the findings for each program evaluation question.
- ☐ Explain and interpret all findings without repeating the results. Why might each finding have occurred? Make sure that each program evaluation question is answered.
- ☐ Explain all unanticipated findings and the occurrence of adverse events as they relate to program risk and safety.
- ☐ In a program evaluation, authors can only state that the program appeared to have effect with the participants. It is important not to overstate findings.
- ☐ Although generalization of the findings from program evaluations cannot be made to the larger population, authors can suggest that the program shows promise and warrants future study with larger sample sizes and more rigorous study methods.
- ☐ Suggest how the program evaluation findings can inform future research needed to build consensus regarding best practice.

Limitations

- ☐ Determine if any of the following weaknesses apply to your program evaluation and should be documented in the Limitations section:
  - ☐ Results may have been biased if multiple facilitators participated in program delivery and varied in the uniformity of program delivery.
  - ☐ Potential bias may have impacted the results if the program facilitator also collected data.
  - ☐ Lack of control and randomization may have biased results because the participants may not represent the larger population.
  - ☐ The possible use of instruments with little or no established psychometric properties may have biased results because it is not clear what such instruments truly measured.
  - ☐ Participant incentives may have biased results because such incentives may have changed participants' motivation for program participation.
  - ☐ Generalization to the larger population cannot be made from a small group of participants.
  - ☐ If follow-up points were not used, it is difficult to understand if patient gains resulting from the program were maintained over time.

Future Directions

- ☐ Describe how future research can address the present program evaluation's limitations.
- ☐ Identify program evaluation questions that remain unanswered and suggest how these questions can be answered in future studies.

Implications for Practice

- ☐ Implications for practice can only relate to the participants in the program and their own clinical course over time. Describe how the present program evaluation's findings can be used to inform clinical decisions for the participants.

- ☐ Describe how the findings from the program evaluation can be used to refine the program for future participants.
- ☐ Describe how findings can be used to design future research with more rigorous methodologies.

Conclusion

- ☐ Summarize the study's primary findings as they relate to (a) the present participants, (b) how findings can be used to refine the program for future participants, and (c) how future research can be designed to assess the program using more rigorous methods.
- ☐ Make sure not to overstate study findings or generalize them to the larger population.

Examples of Well-Written Program Evaluation Journal Articles

Bellum, D., Dahl-Popolizio, S., Bay, R. C., Zhu, A., Fine, J., Kotter, B., Glenn, A., & Wolf, R. L. (2025). Evaluation of an occupational therapy intervention in prisons to prepare incarcerated individuals for successful community reentry. *Open Journal of Occupational Therapy, 13*(2), 1–19. https://doi.org/10.15453/2168-6408.2348

Ham, P. (2025). An academic self-regulation program for first-generation students in occupational therapy: A preexperimental study. *Open Journal of Occupational Therapy, 13*(1), 1–22. https://doi.org/10.15453/2168-6408.2254

Reynolds, L., Buchanan, B., Crabtree, S., & Bordanave, E. (2023). A program to improve the quality of life of caregivers of older adults with chronic conditions: A pilot study. *Open Journal of Occupational Therapy, 11*(2), 1–11. https://doi.org/10.15453/2168-6408.2073

References

American Psychological Association. (2020). *Publication manual of the American Psychological Association* (7th ed.). Author.

Mosey, A. C. (1996). *Applied scientific inquiry in the health professions: An epistemological orientation* (2nd ed.). American Occupational Therapy Association.

CHAPTER 10

Reporting Statistical Data in Text and Tables

Correctly preparing a capstone or research manuscript involves the appropriate reporting of numbers, statistics, symbols, and mathematical copy in text and tables. Inappropriate reporting of these items can adversely influence an editor's, reviewer's, and reader's perception of a manuscript's quality. There are numerous rules guiding the reporting of numbers and statistical data detailed in the *Publication Manual of the American Psychological Association,* 7th ed. (American Psychological Association, 2020). Rather than duplicate this information, this section aims to review the most commonly used rules and help authors avoid frequently made mistakes.

Numbers

- Numbers that immediately precede a unit of measurement should be written in numeric form.
  - 5 mm, 1 in, 6 lb
- Numbers that represent statistical or mathematical functions, percentages, ratios, decimals, and fractions should be written in numeric form.
  - 7% of the population
  - More males than females have a diagnosis of autism spectrum disorder (ASD) at a ratio of 4:1
  - The 3rd percentile
  - 4 times as many adults
- Numbers that represent time, dates, age, and exact monetary sums should be written in numeric form.
  - The test takes 1 hour to administer.
  - The second phase began at 3:00 pm.
  - The patient was 8 years old.
  - Participants were given $5 as an incentive.

DOI: 10.4324/9781003734550-10

Exception: When *approximating* the number of days, months, and years, spell out numbers.
  - The participant had a biopsy approximately two months ago.
- Numbers that represent scores or points on an instrument scale should be written in numeric form.
  - Participant B scored 5 on a 20-point scale.
- Numbers that indicate a place in a series should be written in numeric form.
  - The students were in grade 5.
  - The instruments were set out on table 3.
  - The participants were at reading level 6.
- Numbers that begin a sentence, title, or heading should always be spelled out.
  - Thirty-three percent of the population experiences anxiety.
  - Fifteen students were selected to participate.
- Common fractions in a sentence should be spelled out.
  - One third of the class scored at the highest percentile.
  - Two-thirds of our participants had concomitant disorders.

Numbers Expressed as Plurals

Numbers in plural form are indicated by adding *s* or *es* to the numeral or word without an apostrophe.

- 1960s
- 50s and 100s
- Sixes, sevens, and eights

Decimals

When writing decimals in the text and in tables, use the following rules:

- When the statistic can exceed 1, use a zero before the decimal point.
  - $t = 0.24$
  - $d = 0.14$
- When the statistic cannot exceed 1, do not use a zero before the decimal point.
  - $p = .05$
  - $r = .68$
- For probability levels, report decimals to two or three places.
  - $p = .027$
  - $p = .001$
  - $p = .05$
- For probability levels, report decimals to two or three places.
- Round all other decimals reported in the text and tables to two decimal places.
  - $t = 0.58$
  - $r = .74$

Statistical Symbols

When writing statistical letters expressed as symbols in text and tables, use the following rules:

- Letters used to indicate the names of statistical tests should be italicized.
  - $F(1, 33) = 4.43, p = .04$, 95% CI [.42, .50]
  - $t = 2.28, p = .032$, 95% CI [.75, .95]
- Use the word, instead of the symbol, when reporting a statistical term in a narrative sentence, but not within parentheses.
  - The mean age was 55 (not the *M* age was 55).
  - Participants ranged in age from 45-65 ($M = 55$, $SD = 10$).

Symbols for Number of Participants

- An uppercase, italicized *N* should be used to indicate the total number of participants for a sample.
  - $N = 50$
- A lowercase, italicized *n* is used to indicate the number of participants in a sample subgroup.
  - $n = 15$

Percent Symbol

- Use the percent symbol when it is preceded by a numeral.
  - 18%
- When a percentage is not preceded by a numeral, spell the word.
  - The percentage of adults with attention-deficit hyperactivity disorder (ADHD) is anticipated to be higher than thought.
- Use the percent symbol, %, in table headings and figure legends to conserve space.
  - Correlation between school drop-out and % of students using alcohol

Spacing of Statistical and Numerical Symbols

Space statistical and numerical symbols as words with typed intervals between symbols and numerals.

- $t = 2.28, p = .032$, 95% CI [.75, .95]
- $F(1, 99) = 6.83, p = .006$, 95% CI [.14, .59]

Reporting Statistical Test Findings in the Results Section

The Results section should contain a reporting of findings in both narrative and statistical symbols and numerals.

- An independent *t*-test found a statistically significant difference between intervention and control groups at 1 month after intervention with a moderate effect size ($t = 3.25$,

$p = .023$, $d = 0.54$, 95% CI [.12, 1.73]). The difference between intervention and control group scores at 6 months after intervention was also statistically significant with a larger effect size ($t = 4.88$, $p = .003$, $d = .89$, 95% CI [1.2, 3.5]).

Reporting Statistical Test Findings in Tables

Statistical data reported in the Results narrative should not be duplicated in tables. Tables show numerical values and text in ordered columns and rows and should be used to present a large amount of data that can only be summarized in the Results narrative. Tables should supplement the Results narrative and provide the data necessary for readers to evaluate the researcher's findings using the study's data set. For example, data such as participant mean scores and standard deviations for several instruments could be efficiently displayed in a table without having to use space in the Results narrative.

Authors should refer to all tables in the Results narrative.

- "Table 1 shows participant mean scores and standard deviations for each performance measure."
- "Participant mean scores indicate that as a group, participant performance was highest on the Global Motor Assessment (see Table 1)."

Tables should be numbered according to the order in which they are referred to in the text.

- Tables begin with "1" and are numbered consecutively.
- Suffixes (Table 5a and 5b) are not used.

Tables should be edited with precision, and visual characteristics should be precise, clear, and easy to understand.

- Make sure that table information matches that reported in the manuscript abstract and text—such as final sample size, sample size of subgroups, and reported statistics.
- Make sure that table column numbers and percentages add up correctly.

Inconsistencies between the manuscript text and tables reflect poorly on manuscript quality.

The American Psychological Association (2020) provides extensive information about table formatting, and we encourage authors to review this information when preparing manuscript tables.

Many journals have a limit on the number of tables that can be submitted in one manuscript, and authors should check a journal's author guidelines to determine table requirements.

Reference

American Psychological Association. (2020). *Publication manual of the American Psychological Association* (7th ed.). Author.

CHAPTER 11

Writing Scholarly Discussion Papers for Publication

A discussion paper is a form of refereed journal article in which the author analyzes a professional controversy and argues for a specific resolution. Many authors confuse opinion papers with scholarly discussion papers. A discussion paper analyzes the body of literature about a specific professional controversy and proposes resolutions supported by an analysis of scholarship and research. A discussion paper is a balanced consideration and presentation of all sides of an argument. In contrast, an opinion paper is a one-sided presentation of the author's personal opinions about a professional issue, may not involve rigorous analysis of literature, and may base proposed resolutions on personal agendas rather than a neutral consideration of the literature and stakeholder needs. As with all scholarly writing, the tone of a discussion paper should be neutral. Discussion papers are appropriate for refereed scholarly journals that publish such columns. Authors are encouraged to refer to a journal's author guidelines to determine whether discussion papers are considered for review.

Topic Selection

Discussion papers address controversies or professional problems whose resolutions will influence the evolution of the profession. A controversy is a dispute about the way in which a problem should be resolved by the profession. Many authors inaccurately think that a discussion paper is an exploration of a current topic that may hold importance to the profession, but has a clear resolution and is not considered controversial. For example, a discussion of the need to increase the diversity (i.e., race or ethnicity, gender, age) of occupational therapists is not a debated controversy and has a clear resolution. The need to increase the diversity of occupational therapists is supported by the American Occupational Therapy Association (2025) and can be achieved by enhancing the diversity of students entering occupational therapy education programs. Examples

DOI: 10.4324/9781003734550-11

of currently debated controversies are (a) the degree required for entry-level occupational therapy practice, (b) whether the American Council for Occupational Therapy Education should require standards regarding academic educational skills for an entry-level occupational therapy degree, and (c) the amount and type of activities that can be credited toward continuing education needed to maintain licensure. These examples of controversies are currently debated by occupational therapists and presently have no clear resolution. Authors who wish to write discussion papers that contribute to the literature should select topics of professional controversy. Current topics that have a clear resolution, while enhancing awareness of an issue, do not substantially contribute to the literature and the evolution of a profession.

Examples of Current Topics That Are Not Professional Controversies

- The need to enhance multicultural competence of occupational therapists
- The need to enhance health literacy of occupational therapy patient information and education
- The need for occupational therapists to develop client-centered assessments and interventions that match the health care goals and values of patients

The above topics hold importance to all occupational therapists but are not debated controversies. Arguments against the above are difficult to imagine. Although the above topics may not be appropriate for refereed journal articles, they would be appropriate for health magazines, newsletters, and official national association position papers.

Examples of Professional Controversies

- The need for specialty certification within occupational therapy and the criteria to attain and maintain such certification
- Whether and to what degree the use of physical agents (e.g., ultrasound, electrical stimulation, shortwave diathermy, dry needling) should be within the practice domain of occupational therapists
- Whether occupational therapy services should require a physician prescription
- The accepted labels with which we identify ourselves (e.g., occupational therapist, occupational therapy assistant, occupational therapy practitioner)

These are currently debated controversies having unclear resolutions and would be appropriate discussion paper topics for refereed journal articles.

Basic Content and Structure of Discussion Papers

Discussion papers are approximately 3,000 words in length and have three primary sections. Authors should refer to a specific journal's author guidelines for instructions to write discussion papers. The following sections should be equally weighted and similar in length.

1. Background of the Controversy
2. Presentation of Arguments for and Against the Controversy
3. Directions for Action

Background of the Controversy

Authors should begin discussion papers by describing the controversy and providing background information. The following questions should be answered:

- What is the controversy?
- What is the historical background of the controversy?
- Who are the stakeholders and what are their interests in the controversy and its resolution?
- What is the impact of the controversy on the involved patient population, profession, and larger society?

This section should be based on current literature and use multiple citations.

Presentation of Arguments for and against the Controversy

In this section, authors should present all arguments or viewpoints of the controversial issue using neutral and unbiased language. The following questions should be answered:

- What are the views of all stakeholders?
- What are all sides of the arguments for and against the controversial issue?
- What are proposed resolutions?
- How will all stakeholders be affected by the controversial issue and proposed resolutions?
- What are the authors' views and why? What resolutions do the authors propose and why?

Answers to the above questions should be based on the literature with multiple citations; authors' original ideas and positions, however, do not require citation. It is important that this section be presented as an unbiased and thorough examination of the controversial issue using neutral language.

Directions for Action

In this section, authors should outline the steps that the profession, or professional groups, must take to promote positive resolution of the controversy. These ideas will largely be generated by the authors and do not need to be derived from previous literature and cited. Citations in this section are often minimal. Neutral, unbiased language should be maintained. This section should be written in full narrative paragraphs (as opposed to bulleted phrases).

Tone

As mentioned above, language in discussion papers should be neutral and unbiased. While it is appropriate for opinion papers to use language that is slanted and passionate, authors of scholarly discussion papers to be published in refereed journals must present an impartial analysis and resolution of the controversial issue. While authors are encouraged to use active voice, they should remember that a discussion paper is not an opinion paper based on personal thoughts and perceptions.

Writing Exercises for Discussion Papers

- Write one sentence that explains the controversy that you are addressing in your discussion paper.
- Provide definitions for each concept or any sub-concepts related to the problem addressed.
- Identify when the problem began and discuss any attempts that have been made to solve the problem and the results of those attempts. Provide citations.
- List the people impacted by the problem and list the people, institutions, or policies that could be involved in solving the problem.

Example of the Development of a Discussion Paper

To illustrate how a discussion paper can be drafted, I will present an editorial that I wrote as editor-in-chief of the *Open Journal of Occupational Therapy* (Dirette, 2021). The editorial was written to discuss the concept of compassion, and how it is defined, taught, and manifested in the profession of occupational therapy. Although the paper is written as an editorial, it still possesses many of the components of a discussion paper; however, it is shorter, and the arguments are less fully developed. At the time I wrote this discussion paper, there was a focus on the concept of grit and some attempts to measure grit in applicants to occupational therapy programs. In response, I address this controversy by explaining how the profession can better identify compassion compared to other concepts, such as sympathy, empathy, and grit; identify and admit students to programs who possess compassion; and teach students and therapists to use compassion in practice.

Compassion: Importance and Implications for the Profession of Occupational Therapy

> The controversy addresses how the profession can better identify compassion compared to other concepts, such as sympathy and empathy. The paper begins with a statement addressing this controversy, followed by definitions of the relevant terminology.

The quote "Be kind; everyone you meet is fighting a hard battle" has been attributed to various sources, including Ian McClaren, Plato, Philo of Alexandria, and John Watson (Quoteresearch, 2010). Although the author is debated, this quote, and similar expressions, have become part of the common vernacular in our culture and are seen often in memes posted on social media. At the core of these expressions is the concept of compassion. But what is compassion, and how is it manifested in the profession of occupational therapy?

Various terms, such as empathy and sympathy, are used, sometimes interchangeably, in relation to compassion, but there are differences in their meaning and ultimately in the resulting actions related to each of these concepts. Empathy is the ability to live vicariously in the emotions, thoughts, and experiences of another person. The term empathy originated from the German word Einfuhlung, which means "feeling in." Empathy is different from sympathy. Sympathy is comprehending the feelings of another, but maintaining an emotional distance that is seen as superior to the other. In a short YouTube animation on empathy, Brené Brown illustrates sympathy as seeing someone in a deep hole, but staying on higher ground and talking above them (Brown, 2016). Whereas empathy is like climbing into the hole, sitting beside the person, making yourself vulnerable to sincerely connect with them, and recognizing their struggle without minimizing it.

Empathy can be further broken down into three types: emotional (affective) empathy, cognitive empathy, and compassion. There is evidence of varied neurological correlates that support this conceptualization, and each of these types leads to different behaviors (Klimecki et al., 2014; Stevens & Taber, 2021).

Here, I further delineate the types of compassion, the neurological correlates, and the behaviors related to each type to provide a neutral basis for understanding these concepts.

Emotional Empathy

Emotional empathy, also referred to as affective empathy, is vicarious feelings related to the other person's emotions (Dor-Ziderman et al., 2021). It is feeling physically along with another person, as though their emotions were contagious, and results in an emotional and physical reaction. Physically, emotional empathy results in a distress reaction for the caregiver with increased autonomic responses (e.g., increased heart rate, sweating) and facial expressions that indicate emotional pain (Dor-Ziderman et al., 2021). The neurological correlates are located in the somatosensory regions and the affective brain circuits; specifically, the anterior/mid cingulate cortex and the anterior insula (Dor-Ziderman et al., 2021; Gu et al., 2013). These areas of the brain are associated with interpreting someone else's pain as your own (Stevens & Taber, 2021). Mirror neurons and oxytocin levels in the brain have also been associated with emotional empathy (Stevens & Taber, 2021).

Because the person is feeling the emotions of the other person, emotional empathy leads to actions to alleviate one's own negative emotions and the suffering of the self. These actions, however, may only alleviate the suffering of the self and not of the other person. Ultimately, the empathetic distress that can be created by emotional empathy may lead to decreased helping behaviors (Eisenberg et al., 1989). For example, after the 2012 school shooting at the Sandy Hook Elementary School in which 26 people were killed, including 20 children, the town of Newton, CT, was overwhelmed with various donations sent by people in memory of the children who died. In all, 65,000 teddy bears, nine tractortrailers full of paper snowflakes, and half a million letters were sent to the town, which then had to find space to warehouse them and personnel to figure out how to manage the piles and piles of inventory (Kix, 2015). These actions, based in emotional empathy, may have alleviated the emotions of the people who sent them, but they did very little for the families who were suffering.

Cognitive Empathy

Cognitive empathy is the ability to know and understand how the other person must feel and think and to analyze the problem. For the individual, this is accomplished through thoughts and understanding. The neurological correlates for cognitive empathy include the dorsomedial prefrontal cortex, the ventromedial prefrontal cortex, the temporoparietal junction, the superior temporal sulcus, the temporal pole, and the inferior frontal gyrus (Stevens & Taber, 2021). These areas of the frontal lobes are associated with higher level reasoning and the ability to distinguish one's self from another person and to interpret others' emotional expressions.

Cognitive empathy leads to problem-solving in which the person takes actions to try to alleviate the pain of the one who is suffering. It may, however, neglect or minimize the distressing emotions of the other person to focus on removing the problem that is causing the distress. In addition, cognitive empathy, when not combined with emotional empathy, can lead to detrimental actions. For example, psychopaths can have cognitive empathy, but typically use it to understand how someone is feeling so that they can use it to manipulate them. They do this without the emotional empathy needed to have regard for how their behaviors make the person feel (Stevens & Taber, 2021).

Compassion

Compassion is feelings of concern for the suffering of others with consideration for both the felt senses and the intellectual situation of the other person without losing one's self. It is feeling and understanding the person's situation with mindfulness, caring, and emotional self-management. Compassion uses emotional intelligence to respond effectively to the situation with loving detachment. The neurological correlates for compassion are associated with higher-order cognitive mechanisms and are linked to motivational circuits or the dopaminergic reward system that increases altruism, helping, and affiliative bonding (Dor-Ziderman et al., 2021). The specific areas include the ventral striatum, the subgenual anterior cingulate cortex, and the medial orbitofrontal cortex (Stevens & Tabor, 2021). These areas of the brain are associated with empathetic concern, reward, pleasure, and pro-social behaviors.

A person's actions that are motivated by compassion are balanced between emotional and cognitive empathy and enable the person to feel and understand the needs of others and to act without becoming overwhelmed with feelings (emotional) or impulsively focused on problem-solving (cognitive). Research has shown that compassionate caring does not result in a person sharing the other's negative feelings, but instead in regulated autonomic responses (e.g., reduced heart rate) and parasympathetic regulatory responses (Dor-Ziderman et al., 2021). Through the comprehension of the others' feelings and an understanding of others' needs, the person takes action to alleviate the suffering of others. These actions include helpfulness, wisdom, warmth, and resolve that together manifest as altruism.

Here, I discuss the social/political context, the people impacted by social injustice, the connection to compassion, and the role of the profession of occupational therapy.

↙

Compassion in Society

The Dalai Lama (1391–1474) said "Love and compassion are necessities, not luxuries. Without them humanity cannot survive" (Quote Master, n.d.). The major social justice, political, environmental, and health events of the past few years have heightened the need for compassion in society. The mistreatment of marginalized groups has stirred a collective social outcry and brought about movements such as Black Lives Matter; Me Too; and the lesbian, gay, bisexual, and transgender (LGBT) equal rights movements. Environmental disasters, such as floods, wildfires, and hurricanes, are on the rise sparking calls for legislation. And the spread of the COVID-19 virus brought political divide, false blame, and discrimination against people from Asian countries. Although they have been divisive, to some extent, these events also have produced compassion for others and have fostered pro-social behaviors in individuals and groups.

Pro-social behaviors, also known as altruism, are acts that are done with selfless concern for others (Stevens & Taber, 2021). Pro-social behaviors result from compassion and serve to alleviate the suffering of others. They are not superficial gestures or virtue signaling, such as wearing ribbons or creating social media posts, most closely associated with emotional empathy, but are acts that try to solve the problems of others through an understanding of what it must be like to be the other person.

The profession of occupational therapy has a history of taking action to respond compassionately to people who are marginalized in society. For example, Peloquin (1990) eloquently framed the profession's response to the acquired immunodeficiency syndrome (AIDS) crisis, and these words are applicable to the major societal issues we currently face. She stated:

> We can let AIDS soften our hearts so that we can be warm and tender with our patients. We can respond with common decency, believing that our collective destiny depends on our response to such a major challenge as AIDS. We can rise above ourselves. We can unite to help the person with AIDS enhance his or her life and, if necessary, face his or her death. As occupational therapists who are often part of the shrinking circle of caregivers for the person with AIDS, we can commit to compassion as we provide appropriate treatment.
>
> *(Peloquin, 1990, p. 277)*

In the next section, I discuss the importance of compassion in occupational therapy education. Students and faculty are identified as stakeholders and potential proponents of compassion. In addition, I begin to identify some potential solutions to the development of compassion in the profession of occupational therapy.

Compassion in Education

Compassion also plays an important role in occupational therapy education. The capacity for compassion needs to be evident in the students we admit to occupational therapy programs. Compassion must be role-modeled and fostered in the students throughout the educational process. And compassion for our students is necessary for feeling and understanding what they require throughout this learning process.

In the introduction to the 25th anniversary edition of the book *Emotional Intelligence: Why it Can Matter More Than IQ*, Goleman (2020) states that the current focus on the concept of grit lacks consideration for compassion and social skills. Grit is achievement and the capacity to overcome personal adversity, but the focus is on the self and not on the much-needed skill of a therapist to focus on others. Grit is somewhat the opposite of compassion. Instead of focusing on grit, there are various ways that occupational therapy programs can take steps to admit students who have the capacity for compassion. One way is to screen students who apply to the program for their capacity for compassion. Gutman and Falk-Kessler (2016) developed and examined the psychometric properties of the Emotional Intelligence (EI) Admission Essay scale for specific use in occupational therapy programs. The moderate to strong psychometric properties suggest that the scale has the ability to provide information about applicants' EI, a concept that is very closely aligned with compassion.

Once students are admitted to an occupational therapy program, steps also can be taken to foster the growth of compassion. There is evidence that compassion training can reduce empathetic distress and strengthen resilience (Klimecki et al., 2014). Several publications in the Topics in Education category in past issues of the *Open Journal of Occupational Therapy* (*OJOT*) have focused on this process. Simulations that help students understand the perspective of the client (Ozelie et al., 2018), clients as presenters to build comfort and understanding (Hedge et al., 2015), and peer-support dyads in challenging fieldworks (Raphael-Greenfield et al., 2017), have all been examined as a means to improve students' level of compassion and success. In addition, Gutman et al. (2020) provided evidence for using multimodal mindfulness as a means for improving self-compassion in occupational and physical therapy students.

Compassion from faculty is also necessary for helping students learn to be occupational therapists. Faculty with backgrounds or generations that are different from their students should use compassion for the perspectives of the students to enhance the learning experience. For example, in a previous issue of *OJOT*, DeIulius and Saylor (2021) explored what helps occupational therapy students from Generations Y and Z to learn. They found that teaching based on coaching and growth mindset philosophies with an emphasis on practice-ready skills and human relationships using guided discovery and modeling enhanced the students' self-awareness and their ability to learn healthy, productive collaboration, workplace etiquette and culture, and ultimately enhanced client-provider relationships.

In the next section, I discuss compassion in occupational therapy practice, examining how it is manifested and how other concepts, such as emotional empathy and sympathy, can be less therapeutically effective. I end this section with two examples to help the reader understand the application of the concept of compassion.

Compassionate Care in Occupational Therapy Practice

Compassionate care in occupational therapy practice is essential for forming therapeutic relationships, problem-solving from the perspective of the client, and providing care that maintains the dignity of the people we serve. According to Peloquin (1995), the therapeutic relationship is based in compassion, and does not "exact a fusion but a connection" (p. 26). The therapeutic relationship is characterized by "an expression of being there, a soul turning, a recognition of likeness and difference, a participation in the experience of another, a connection with feeling, a power to recover from that connection, and a personal enrichment" (Peloquin, 1995, p. 30–31). She states that therapists must have the capacity to apprehend, imagine, and feel and that they must convey understanding as they strive to solve heath care problems (Peloquin, 1995). Therapists "must know how to be there for their patients, fiercely caring, while standing as themselves" (Peloquin, 1995, p. 26).

While compassion leads to action to alleviate the suffering of others, emotional empathy may lead to empathetic distress and be counterproductive in the therapeutic process. If a therapist is functioning in an emotional empathic mode, they may become overwhelmed, violate professional boundaries, and ultimately become burned out (Klimecki et al., 2014; Sinclair et al., 2017). Furthermore, it was found that clients can distinguish among sympathetic and compassionate care and prefer the latter (Sinclair et al., 2017).

In clinical practice, I have seen compassionate occupational therapy care in action. In one case, our rehabilitation team was completely flummoxed and frustrated by a client who was admitted to our inpatient brain injury rehabilitation unit. The client, a middle-aged man who was a professional choreographer, was refusing to participate in any rehabilitation assessments or interventions. In addition, he was shouting insults and obscenities at anyone who dared enter his hospital room. With fair warning from the nurses, I entered his room, made a request to have him participate in a cognitive assessment, and received my share of his agitation. I left some of the paper forms on his bedside table and left the room. The next day, I walked by his room and, to my surprise, the occupational therapy assistant was sitting next to his bed and the patient was filling out the assessments I had left with him. When she finished, I inquired how she managed to accomplish such a feat. She explained that she was thinking about what his life was like before his brain injury and what it was like now. She had come to the conclusion that he was used to giving orders and now was being told what to do. So, she just entered his room, sat in a chair and said to him, "let me know if you need anything." He first requested a glass of water. Then, he asked for the bed to be adjusted. Next, after she mentioned the paperwork on his bedside table, he told her to give it to him so he could look at it. She did and his response was, "well, if you don't give me a pen, how am I going to fill it out?" She gave him a pen and he filled them out. The compassionate approach of exploring what he was experiencing balanced with an understanding his view of the world lead to the actions that solved the problem in a manner that maintained his dignity.

In another such scenario, I was working at the lunchtime feeding group table in a rehabilitation hospital patient cafeteria. A young man, who was blind from his brain injury, was assigned to the table because he was refusing to eat. He already had been through training on eating hand-held foods, using a spoon and bowl, and drinking from cups, and he had managed this quite well in the privacy of his hospital room. So, my thought was that he might be depressed or embarrassed to eat and drink in the cafeteria. I chatted with him for a bit to get a sense of how he was feeling, but neither of those seemed to be his experience. Next, thinking that he might not know what to order, I read the entire cafeteria menu to him and his response was, "I'll just have a glass of water." When I returned to the table and put the water in his hands, something clicked. I could tell by his response that he thought I was a waitress. It was suddenly apparent to me that he had probably only ever eaten in a hospital cafeteria when visiting the hospital and therefore thought that he had to pay. I explained who I was and that there was no charge for any food or drinks in the hospital patient cafeteria. He then ordered three hamburgers, french fries, and a coke … and he ate all of it! In this situation, a compassionate understanding of his perspective lead to actions to solve the problem in a manner that maintained his dignity. In these, as in many other therapeutic situations that I have witnessed, compassionate caring was at the heart of the interaction. As Peloquin (1995) described, it is "a way of seeing with the eyes of others to appreciate nuances in their visions of the world. To be present for one's patients empathically is to take a stand from which one participates in their experiences" (p. 26).

Because this was an editorial discussion paper, I used this section to connect the concept of compassion to the articles published in that issue of *The Open Journal of Occupational Therapy*. This is not a typical section of a discussion paper, but more likely found in letters from the editor. In a full discussion paper, authors could insert a similar section in which the literature is reviewed to illustrate resolutions to the problems discussed.

In This Issue

While compassion is not the primary topic in any of the articles published in this issue, it is a theme that threads throughout. In this issue, the Applied Research topics are varied and include an exploration of the impact of safe spaces on occupation and well-being for older adults in an LGBT residential community, the development of a model of occupation-based practice, a systematic review on self-advocacy interventions conducted in group and community-based settings, a scoping review of occupational therapy approaches to enable occupations for people living with behavioral disturbance following acquired brain injuries, an evaluation of the content validity of the clinical competency assessment tool for occupational therapists treating patients with neurodegenerative disease, a scoping review of health literacy in occupational therapy practice, and a feasibility study of a Tai Chi program to enhance the quality of life for older adults in assisted living facilities. Each of these research projects provides insight on the perspectives of the people with whom we work and presents evidence for our treatment approaches. In addition, two Guidelines for Practice articles are presented. One guideline is for teaching students with intellectual or developmental disability vocational skills, life skills, activities of daily living, instrumental activities of daily living, and community participation, and the other is to promote social participation in adolescents with burn injuries. In the Topics in Education category, authors discuss research on using simulation-based learning for working in mental health and service learning in primary care. The issue concludes with two Opinions in the Profession articles. One of the articles discusses the role of occupational therapy in meeting the needs of the aging LGBT population, and the other discusses the role of occupational therapy in assisting people to rediscover purpose and promote physical and emotional well-being during the global COVID-19 pandemic.

Here, I provide a conclusion that summarizes the concept and emphasizes the importance of compassion for the stakeholder and for the profession of occupational therapy. Authors should include a conclusion or a summary with final thoughts related to the topic discussed.

↙

Conclusion

In the profession of occupational therapy, we must strive to have compassion and to provide compassionate care. We must have compassion, not just for those who are marginalized by society, but for all people we serve. We must have compassion, not just for people with whom we identify, but for those from whom we are different and for those with whom we disagree. As stated by Albert Schweitzer, "The purpose of human life is to serve, and to show compassion and the will to help others" (Brainy Quote, n.d.). In this, and in all issues of *OJOT*, we endeavor to promote compassionate caring in the profession of occupational therapy. Whether we are discussing social participation for adolescents with burn injuries, occupational therapy interventions for people with behavioral issues following acquired brain injury, or the rights of the aging community who identify as LGBT, compassion is at the core.

The discussion paper should end with references that are formatted according to the author guidelines for the publication to which the discussion paper is submitted.

↙

References

BrainyQuote. (n.d.). *Albert Schweitzer quotes*. www.brainyquote.com/quotes/albert_schweitzer_133530

Brown, B. (2016). *Empathy vs. sympathy* [Video]. YouTube. www.youtube.com/watch?v=KZBTYViDPlQ

DeIuliis, E. D., & Saylor, E. (2021). Bridging the gap: Three strategies to optimize professional relationships with Generation Y and Z. *The Open Journal of Occupational Therapy, 9*(1), 1–13. https://doi.org/10.15453/2168-6408.1748

Dor-Ziderman, Y., Cohen, D., Levit-Binnun, N., & Golland, Y. (2021). Synchrony with distress in affective empathy and compassion. *Psychophysiology, 58*, e13889. https://doi.org/10.1111/psyp.13889

Eisenberg, N., Fabes, R., Miller, P., Fultz, J., Shell, R., Mathy, R., & Reno, R. R. (1989). Relation of sympathy and personal distress to prosocial behaviour: A multimethod study. *Journal of Personality and Social Psychology, 57*(1), 55–66. https://doi.org/10.1037/0022-3514.57.1.55

Goleman, D. (2020). *Emotional intelligence: Why it can matter more than IQ*. Bantam Books.

Gu, X., Hof, P. R., Friston, K. J., & Fan, J. (2013). Anterior insular cortex and emotional awareness. *The Journal of Comparative Neurology, 521*(15), 3371–3388. https://doi.org/10.1002/cne.23368

Gutman, S. A., & Falk-Kessler, J. P. (2016). Development and psychometric properties of the emotional intelligence admission essay scale. *The Open Journal of Occupational Therapy, 4*(3). https://doi.org/10.15453/2168-6408.1233

Gutman, S. A., Sliwinski, M., Laird, J., & Nguyen, J. (2020). Effectiveness of a multimodal mindfulness program for student health care professionals: A randomized controlled trial. *The Open Journal of Occupational Therapy, 8*(2), 1–18. https://doi.org/10.15453/2168-6408.1662

Hedge, N., Neville, M. A., & Pickens, N. D. (2015). How patient educators teach students: "Giving a face to a story." *The Open Journal of Occupational Therapy, 3*(1). https://doi.org/10.15453/2168-6408.1143

Kix, P. (2015). 65,000 teddy bears for Newtown, and one man to sort the world's grief. *The Trace*. www.thetrace.org/2015/12/sandy-hookshooting-donations/

Klimecki, O. M., Leiberg, S., Ricard, M., & Singer, T. (2014). Differential pattern of functional brain plasticity after compassion and empathy training. *Social Cognitive and Affective Neuroscience, 9*(6), 873–879. https://doi.org/10.1093/scan/nst060

Ozelie, R., Panfil, P., Swiderski, N., & Walz, E. (2018). Hearing voices simulation: Impact on occupational therapy students. *The Open Journal of Occupational Therapy, 6*(4). https://doi.org/10.15453/2168-6408.1452

Peloquin, S. M. (1990). AIDS: Toward a compassionate response. *American Journal of Occupational Therapy, 44*(3), 271–278. https://doi.org/10.5014/ajot.44.3.271

Peloquin, S. M. (1995). The fullness of empathy: Reflections and illustrations. *American Journal of Occupational Therapy, 49*(1), 24–31. https://doi.org/10.5014/ajot.49.1.24

Quote Master. (n.d.). *Dalai Lama*. www.quotemaster.org/q1dee9c85a9a606e1339fc7e96932c4ba

Quote Investigator. (2010). *Be kind; everyone you meet is fighting a hard battle*. https://quoteinvestigator.com/2010/06/29/bekind/

Raphael-Greenfield, E., Miranda-Capella, I., & Branch, M. (2017). Adapting to a challenging fieldwork: Understanding the ingredients. *The Open Journal of Occupational Therapy, 5*(1). https://doi.org/10.15453/2168-6408.1257

Sinclair, S., Beamer, K., Hack, T. F., McClement, S., Bouchal, S. R., Chochinov, H. M., & Hagen, N. A. (2017). Sympathy, empathy, and compassion: A grounded theory study of palliative care patients' understandings, experiences, and preferences. *Palliative Medicine, 31*(5), 437–447. https://doi.org/10.1177/0269216316663499

Stevens, F., & Taber, K. (2021). The neuroscience of empathy and compassion in pro-social behavior. *Neuropsychologia, 159*, 107925. https://doi.org/10.1016/j.neuropsychologia.2021.107925

Checklist for Writing a Scholarly Discussion Paper

- ☐ Select a professional controversy.
- ☐ Outline the paper using three primary sections:

1. **Background of the Controversy**
   - ☐ Answer the following questions:
     - ☐ What is the controversy?
     - ☐ What is the historical background of the controversy?
     - ☐ Who are the stakeholders and what are their interests in the controversy and its resolution?
     - ☐ What is the impact of the controversy on the involved patient population, profession, and larger society?
     - ☐ Use the literature and citations.
     - ☐ Keep tone and language neutral.
2. **Arguments For and Against the Controversial Issue**
   - ☐ The following questions should be answered:
     - ☐ What are the views of all stakeholders?
     - ☐ What are all sides of the arguments for and against the controversial issue?
     - ☐ What are proposed resolutions?
     - ☐ How will all stakeholders be affected by the controversial issue and proposed resolutions?
     - ☐ What are the authors' views and why? What resolutions do the authors propose and why?
   - ☐ Use the literature and citations.
   - ☐ Keep tone and language neutral.
3. **Directions for Action**
     - ☐ Present the steps that the profession, or professional groups, must take to promote positive resolution of the controversy.
     - ☐ Because directions for action are based on the authors' ideas, citations in this section will often be minimal.
     - ☐ Maintain neutral language and tone.

References

American Occupational Therapy Association. (2025). Advocacy issues: Supporting a diverse workplace. www.aota.org/advocacy/issues/supporting-a-diverse-workforce#:~:text=The%20American%20Occupational%20Therapy%20Association%20(AOTA)%20advocates,to%20mirror%20the%20makeup%20of%20the%20population

Dirette, D. P. (2021). Compassion: Importance and implications for the profession of occupational therapy. *Open Journal of Occupational Therapy, 9*(4), 1–6. https://doi.org/10.15453/2168-6408.1951

CHAPTER 12

Turning Dissertations, Capstone Theses, and Clinical Data into Publishable Journal Articles

Turning Doctoral Work into Journal Manuscripts

An increasingly popular model for doctoral degree programs requires students to develop three journal articles based on their dissertation or capstone thesis. This requirement helps doctoral students to transform their dissertation or capstone thesis into separate but related journal article manuscripts that can be submitted to various journals. Dissertation and capstone committee members, who may be listed as coauthors in the published work, provide guidance regarding the development of the three journal manuscripts. This model helps students transition from the role of doctoral student to academic author.

Most doctoral degree programs, however, are based on the traditional model in which the student completes novel research or clinical work and reports the results in a lengthy dissertation or capstone thesis. Dissertations and capstone theses can often exceed 100 typed pages and are commonly structured by independent chapters that more aptly resemble a book than a journal article. Students are commonly expected to develop the skills needed to transform a dissertation or capstone thesis from a 100+ page manuscript consisting of multiple chapters into two or three 25-page journal manuscripts on their own.

Returning to Your Research or Project Questions

To begin transforming the dissertation or capstone thesis into several journal articles, authors should return to their research or project questions. Commonly, dissertations and capstone theses involve a novel examination of several clinical questions and subquestions designed to investigate a specific topic. The most efficient way of turning the dissertation or capstone thesis into multiple journal manuscripts is to pull out the primary project questions and structure manuscripts around them.

Let us consider, for example, a doctoral student whose capstone thesis examined the effect of an intervention designed to help homeless adults transition to supportive housing.

DOI: 10.4324/9781003734550-12

Capstone questions consisted of the following:

1. What are the self-identified occupational needs of formerly homeless adults who now reside in supportive housing?
2. How do common physical, cognitive, and mental health problems of this population impact daily function in supportive housing?
3. Can an occupational therapy intervention effectively help formerly homeless adults in supportive housing function better in daily life activities compared to adults in a waitlist control group?

The capstone thesis was divided into the following chapters based on the three project questions above:

1. Introduction: The State of Homelessness in the United States Today
2. Literature Review
    - Who Becomes Homeless and Why?
    - Types of Supportive Housing for Homeless Adults
    - The Role of Occupational Therapy in the Transition to and Maintenance of Supportive Housing
3. Methods
4. Results
    - Self-Identified Occupational Needs of Formerly Homeless Adults Residing in Supportive Housing
    - Physical, Cognitive, and Mental Health Problems of Formerly Homeless Adults that Impact Daily Function in Supportive Housing
    - Effect of an Occupational Therapy Intervention to Help Formerly Homeless Adults Residing in Supportive Housing to Function Better in Daily Life Activities
5. Discussion

This capstone thesis was restructured into three journal manuscripts based on the project questions. Background information about homelessness from the capstone project's introduction and literature review was used in all three articles but reworded in each manuscript to avoid self-plagiarism and violation of journal copyright regulations.

- The first manuscript reported the findings yielded from the following capstone thesis question: What are the self-identified occupational needs of formerly homeless adults who now reside in supportive housing? In this substudy of the capstone thesis, the author used qualitative methods to interview seven male and female adults who were homeless for a range of 3–5 years to determine their self-perceived occupational needs. The author found that the participants, once housed, led isolated lives but wished to better integrate and participate in community life. Desired occupations included volunteerism, joining supportive housing recreational groups, and obtaining employment. Fear of being in the community and lack of foundational educational skills impeded participants' ability to engage in desired occupations. The author used the manuscript formatting guidelines for a general research study in Chapter 4 to revise this specific capstone thesis material into a separate, stand-alone manuscript.

- The second manuscript reported the findings from the following capstone project question: How do common physical, cognitive, and mental health problems of this population impact daily function in supportive housing? To answer this substudy question, the author used a mixed-method design in which qualitative interviewing was used to understand the types of physical, cognitive, and mental health problems participants perceived as impediments to their daily function in supportive housing. The author also used the Westmead Home Safety Assessment (Clemson, Fitzgerald, & Heard, 1999) to perform an environmental evaluation of the supportive housing environment. Participants commonly reported that memory problems (largely from substance use histories and assault) impacted their ability to manage medications and medical appointments and return to school or work. Participants also experienced a range of physical problems—primarily chronic pain—which prevented their participation in community life, hindered their function in the supportive housing apartment, and disrupted sleep. Posttraumatic stress disorder was also experienced by many of the participants, who stated that they had difficulty being in crowds on the subway and city streets and preferred to be alone. The manuscript formatting guidelines for a general research study in Chapter 4 were used to revise this material into a separate, stand-alone manuscript.
- The third manuscript derived from the author's capstone thesis reported the findings from the following project question: Can an occupational therapy intervention effectively help formerly homeless adults in supportive housing function better in daily life activities compared to adults in a waitlist control group? To answer this question, the author nonrandomly divided her convenience sample into two groups: an intervention group of four participants who received the occupational therapy intervention and a waitlist control group of three participants. The intervention consisted of environmental modifications to the home to enhance function and safety in the bathroom, kitchen, and bedroom. Cognitive compensatory strategies were used to help participants with medication management, medical appointment tracking, and money management. After the 3-month intervention, participants in the intervention group reported enhanced function in the supportive housing environment (e.g., being able to rise from the bed and toilet more easily) and had lowered their incidence of forgetting to take medication or attend medical appointments. Participants in the waitlist control group did not show the same improvement in safety and function. The author used the manuscript formatting guidelines for intervention effectiveness studies in Chapter 5 to revise this material into a separate, stand-alone manuscript.
- A fourth journal article could have reported the details of one participant's intervention experience in a case report format. Using the guidelines for case reports in Chapter 8, the author could have illustrated the characteristics of the intervention by describing the participant's baseline, intervention, and postintervention functional activity status.

When authors develop separate, stand-alone journal manuscripts from their dissertation or capstone thesis as novice writers, it is important to seek feedback from seasoned academic writers. If feedback and revision offered by mentors is significant, mentors may be offered coauthorship to ready the manuscript for publication. Working with mentors to develop separate journal articles from the dissertation or capstone thesis is a valuable learning experience and can help novice writers learn academic writing skills.

Commonly Made Mistakes in the Transformation of Dissertations and Capstone Theses into Journal Articles

One commonly made mistake that novice authors make when transforming their dissertation or capstone thesis into separate journal manuscripts is to submit dissertation or thesis chapters without revising them in accordance with reporting standards and journal author guidelines. Sometimes authors cut and paste pieces from the original dissertation or thesis without attempting to reformat the work into a cohesive and logically flowing journal manuscript. Authors must remember that the dissertation and thesis have distinct requirements and objectives that differ from those of a journal manuscript. Dissertations and theses are required to adhere to the style guidelines of a specific university rather than a journal. Students sometimes make the mistake of believing that the research procedures and style guidelines taught by their university mentors are the only correct methods and do not consider the need to revise before submitting to a journal. It is imperative to seek the author guidelines of specific journals to which authors wish to submit and revise doctoral work in accordance with those guidelines. It is also critical to use the reporting standards for specific types of research studies to transform doctoral work into publishable journal articles.

It is essential that authors transform their dissertations or theses into publishable journal manuscripts as quickly as possible after the completion of doctoral work. Too often, authors make the mistake of accepting faculty positions, clinical appointments, or engaging in family and life events, and allow too much time to elapse after doctoral degree completion. Soon the dissertation or thesis becomes abandoned as more time passes and authors become involved in other activities. Failing to transform the dissertation or thesis into two or more journal articles is a lost opportunity because the data have been collected and analyzed. Having access to collected and analyzed data that are ready to be developed into one or more journal manuscripts will never occur as readily again.

Turning Doctoral Degree Class Assignments into Publishable Discussion Papers

Occasionally doctoral students take courses in which they complete paper assignments that they later wish to transform into a publishable discussion paper addressing a professional issue. When doctoral students wish to turn their class paper assignments into discussion papers for publication, it is essential to revise the paper into a journal manuscript that matches a specific journal's publication goals and style guidelines. Some authors make the mistake of submitting paper assignments as originally written or do not read the journal's author guidelines to determine whether a paper topic and format are congruent with the journal's publication objectives. Authors wishing to revise coursework into publishable discussion papers should read Chapter 11, Writing Scholarly Discussion Papers for Publication.

Checklist for Turning Doctoral Work into Journal Submissions

- ☐ To transform dissertation and thesis work into journal manuscripts, take the primary research or project questions and structure manuscripts around them.
- ☐ Although authors can use material from the dissertation or thesis introduction and literature review as background information in multiple journal manuscripts, the wording should be altered in each manuscript to avoid self-plagiarism and copyright violations.
- ☐ Identify the types of journal manuscripts (e.g., general research manuscript, intervention effectiveness manuscript, instrument development and testing manuscript, case report manuscript, or discussion paper manuscript) you will develop from the dissertation or thesis and use the reporting standards in this book as formatting guides.
- ☐ Identify journals whose publication objectives correspond to your project and obtain their author guidelines. Use the author guidelines to determine such things as the appropriate style guide and limitations on the number of references, tables, figures, and words.
- ☐ Seek feedback on manuscript drafts from seasoned academic writers. Consider inviting seasoned academic writers to become coauthors to make revisions needed for journal submission readiness.
- ☐ Do not submit dissertation or thesis chapters as originally written without making modifications needed for journal submission.
- ☐ Do not cut and paste original pieces from the dissertation or thesis without attempting to rewrite the manuscript into a cohesive and logically flowing stand-alone paper. Cutting and pasting pieces from the original doctoral work into a journal manuscript will make the manuscript appear disjointed, poorly organized, and lacking continuity.
- ☐ Transform the dissertation or thesis into publishable journal articles as quickly as possible after completing doctoral work. The longer authors wait to publish articles from their doctoral work, the less likely they will be to accomplish this achievement.
- ☐ To transform a class assignment into a publishable discussion paper, authors should revise their writing in accordance with the author guidelines of a specific journal to which they wish to submit. Do not submit the assignment as originally written for a specific class. Make sure that the journal to which you wish to submit publishes discussion papers similar to yours.

Turning Clinical Data into Possible Journal Articles

Retrospective Studies

Clinicians have access to patients and patient databases and can often formulate fundamental and relevant clinical research questions about evaluation and treatment practices. The collaboration between clinicians and researchers is a vital one needed to ask and answer the most critical questions about clinical practice. Clinicians who wish to participate in research but do not have specific, well-defined research questions should contact occupational therapy academic faculty and researchers to determine whether collaborative research can be developed based on the clinical database to which practitioners have access. In this context, a retrospective research study can be designed in which a research question is asked and answered using already collected patient data that will be de-identified to protect patient anonymity and confidentiality. For example, a clinician may work with patients who have moderate spasticity in their upper extremities resulting from neurologic insult. A research study could be formulated that examines the effectiveness of two different types of splints. The patient database could be used to examine functional outcomes of similar patients who received splint A compared to splint B.

In another example of the use of retrospectively collected data, a clinician in the school system may work with second graders with handwriting deficits identified by teachers. The database could be used to examine the effectiveness of handwriting interventions that were provided (a) in the classroom in a group format or (b) in one-to-one pullout sessions with the child and therapist.

Although retrospective studies require institutional review board approval, they may be easier to conduct than prospective studies because they do not require participant recruitment; participant and/or guardian consent; and anonymization procedures for recruiters, interveners, data collectors, and data analysts. These elements of prospective studies enhance design rigor but are more difficult to implement. Often clinicians who participate in prospective studies do so as data collectors in collaboration with principal investigators who are able to oversee study design formulation, institutional review board approval, participant recruitment and consent, anonymization procedures, intervention fidelity measurement, data analysis, and dissemination of results. Clinicians who wish to participate in prospective studies should contact health care academic faculty and researchers at regional institutions of higher learning to determine whether collaboration is possible.

Case Reports or Case Series

The reporting of novel intervention through case reports or case series is a form of retrospective research that can be easily accomplished by clinicians who have provided treatment. Because case reports and case series only address one to three patients' treatment experience, it is easier to accomplish than retrospective studies having larger databases. In the case report or case series, occupational therapists have usually provided unique intervention to one to three patients having positive outcomes. The intervention may show promise of helping more patients with similar clinical conditions, and thus the reported findings are disseminated to the clinical community. For example, a therapist may document the intervention provided to a patient with traumatic brain injury who has significant visual-perceptual deficits. The case report addresses patient history, intervention description, baseline measures, postintervention outcomes, and patient satisfaction. Although Chapter 8 provides details about the formatting necessary for writing a case report manuscript, we recommend that therapists who are not comfortable with academic journal writing seek mentorship from a seasoned academic writer. An academic writer may be offered coauthorship if they significantly contribute to the writing of the final manuscript, which may be necessary for manuscript publication readiness.

Checklist for Turning Clinical Data into Possible Research Studies

- ☐ Determine whether as a clinician you have access to a specific patient database and what type of information is provided in that database (e.g., patient demographics, clinical conditions, intervention, outcomes).
- ☐ Determine whether you have specific clinical questions about evaluation and practice that can be answered through a retrospective examination of your patient database or if a seasoned researcher and faculty member can help you formulate clinical questions.
- ☐ Contact and meet with seasoned researchers to refine research questions, develop study procedures, seek institutional review board approval, implement study procedures, collect data, analyze data, and report written results using an appropriate manuscript reporting standard format.
- ☐ Determine whether as a clinician you have a unique patient case that can be turned into a case report or case series for publication.
- ☐ Determine whether the intervention provided is novel or if the patient's clinical condition has not been previously addressed by the profession and documented in the literature.
- ☐ Make sure that you have collected baseline and postintervention measurements using standardized instruments.
- ☐ If you do not feel comfortable with the academic writing skills needed to construct a case report or case series manuscript for publication (as described in Chapter 8), seek help from a seasoned academic researcher or faculty member. If this professional assumes a significant portion of the writing, coauthorship should be negotiated.

Reference

Clemson, L., Fitzgerald, M. H., & Heard, R. (1999). Content validity of an assessment tool to identify home fall hazards: The Westmead Home Safety Assessment. *British Journal of Occupational Therapy*, *62*(4), 171–179. https://doi.org/10.1177/030802269906200407

CHAPTER 13

The Publication Process

Preparing and Submitting Manuscripts for Publication

All journals have author guidelines that provide instructions for the preparation and submission of manuscripts. Readers are encouraged to obtain and adhere to the guidelines of the specific journal to which they wish to submit at an early stage in the manuscript development process. This section helps readers understand the process of preparing manuscripts for submission and publication.

Authorship and Corresponding Author Responsibilities

Authorship is the assignment of ownership of a piece of written scholarship. Chapter 17 reviews the ethical considerations of authorship and provides guidelines for establishing author identification and order. At the time of submission, author identification and order should have been established. The first author, the author who has made the most substantial contributions to a study, is commonly but not always, the corresponding author. The corresponding author is the author who assumes responsibility for manuscript final preparation before submission, manuscript submission, all resubmissions, and all correspondence with the editor. It is the corresponding author's responsibility to ensure that the manuscript is prepared in accordance with author guidelines, that resubmissions thoroughly address requested revisions by editors and reviewers, that page proofs are correct and accurately reflect authors' work, and that copyright forms are correctly signed and submitted by all authors (or as required by a specific journal). Some journals provide the email address of the corresponding author so that researchers can contact this author about study content.

Journal Selection

After authors have collected, analyzed, and interpreted data and are ready to write the manuscript narrative, they should begin to formulate ideas about the type of journals that best match their completed research. It is good practice to select two

DOI: 10.4324/9781003734550-13

to three possible journals and rank each journal's congruence with your study. Most journals describe commonly published article types and publication goals in their author guidelines. Because dual or simultaneous submission to two or more journals is considered publication misconduct, authors should select one journal and use that journal's author guidelines to prepare and format their manuscript. Author guidelines can be easily located on a journal's website. Do not assume that you are familiar with a specific journal's author guidelines and fail to obtain them. Journals update author guidelines frequently, particularly as a result of changing copyright laws and new and revised reporting guidelines.

Following Author Guidelines and Formatting Styles

Once you have obtained the author guidelines for the journal to which you wish to submit, it is important to read the entire narrative and make notes about essential points, including the following:

- Page length requirements for the entire manuscript
- Word count requirements for the entire manuscript
- Spacing of type
- Font type and size
- Margin size
- Page numbering
- Abstract word count
- Abstract headings
- Use of key words
- Table and figure count limitations
- Requirements concerning permission to reprint published materials
- Masking procedures

Author guidelines will state which style guide should be used by authors to format manuscripts. In the health professions, many journals use the *Publication Manual of the American Psychological Association*, 7th ed. (American Psychological Association, 2020). Authors should obtain the indicated style guide and ensure that their manuscript adheres to style guide specifications; detailed attention should be paid to citation and reference formatting. Software programs are available that can convert references into a variety of style guide formats. Manuscripts that do not adhere to a journal's author guidelines and designated style guide format reflect poorly on a submission. Such manuscripts appear to have been previously submitted to and rejected by another journal. Manuscripts with numerous style guide and author guideline errors are more difficult for editors and reviewers to evaluate.

Manuscript Masking

Most journals request that a masked manuscript be submitted alone or in addition to an unmasked copy. Masking means that all identifying author information (including names and affiliations) and institution names (i.e., the names of universities and clinical facilities) be removed from the manuscript. The acknowledgment section should also be removed from a masked manuscript copy. Using masked manuscripts in the review process enhances confidentiality and promotes ethical review processes. Commonly overlooked items that should be masked include the institutional review board's affiliated university name, the names of clinical facilities from which participants were recruited, and the authors' names in manuscript citations and references. Participant identities should never be revealed through manuscript photographs or by naming the clinical facility at which they received treatment.

Writing Concisely and Precisely

Many authors contact editors to justify why their papers should be published in excess of page length limitations. Such justifications usually address the significance of findings and the need to publish all results in one paper. There is never a defensible reason why a paper must be published in excess of page length requirements. If a paper is significantly over length, it should be revised into two separate papers. A paper that is moderately over length should be edited for conciseness. Authors should consider the following:

- Whether all tables/figures are essential or can be deleted or reduced in size
- Whether the literature addresses the focused topic or extends beyond material necessary to describe background information
- Whether the Discussion section is concise and conveys the simplest interpretation of findings or extends beyond study results

In many submissions, the Method section is not adequately described in accordance with transparent reporting standards and requires additional information. Key sections most commonly requiring editing to reduce length are the Introduction (and embedded literature review) and Discussion. Many manuscripts contain information in the Introduction and Discussion sections that is extraneous to the study presentation and can be removed. Authors must seek to write concisely and precisely—that is, formulate sentences conveying the greatest amount of meaning while using the least amount of words. Writing concisely and precisely is a learned skill that can be enhanced through writing practice, multiple paper revisions, and working with a competent editor who can edit papers for clarity, reduced length, and word choice precision. Such editors are commonly employed by authors for personal use; it is not the responsibility of journal editor-in-chiefs to assist with major manuscript editing. Writing concisely and precisely most clearly conveys the author's intended message to readers. The focused message of a manuscript should be described using simple language that is not lost in technical jargon and long discourses. Concise and precise language can be facilitated by the use of active voice. While traditional journal writing has encouraged authors to use third-person language, most journals now require authors to use active voice in an effort to enhance transparency of research procedures and researcher roles.

Writing without Bias

Writing without bias involves presenting written ideas without prejudice or disposition regarding gender, sex, sexual orientation, race and ethnicity, disability, and age.

Minimal reporting standards mandate that the participant demographics of sex, race/ethnicity, disability, and age should always be reported to promote transparency and reduce bias in research studies. This section provides guidance for authors to both identify and remove bias from written scholarship.

Gender, Sex, and Sexual Orientation

Gender is the cultural interpretation of male and female roles and is self-assigned based on the individual's personal feelings about being male or female in a particular social group (Rothenberg, 2013). Sex is the biological designation of male or female based on genetics and the appearance of reproductive organs. With gender reassignment surgery, mixed phenotype births (e.g., both male and female reproductive organs may be present), and a variety of chromosomal patterns (in which a phenotypic male may appear female and vice versa), sex assignment can be unclear and should be designated by study participants rather than researchers.

Sexual orientation is the self-identified attraction to males, females, or both (Conron, Mimiaga, & Landers, 2010) and should also be designated by participants rather than researchers. Unless your study specifically addresses sexual orientation as a variable that impacts results and data interpretation, sexual orientation should not be reported as a participant demographic. The reporting of sexual orientation when this demographic does not impact study findings is biased and implies that people with differing sexual orientations have innate differences from others beyond sexual attraction.

When reporting sex of participants, do not report one sex's n value without reporting the other's. For example, "There were 39 participants (male = 17)." Instead, report both: "There were 39 participants (male = 17; female = 22)." Reporting the number of only one group implies that the other group's data are unimportant.

Both sexes collectively should not be referred to as *mankind* or *man*; *humans* or *people* can be used instead. The pronoun *he* should not be used to refer to both sexes. For example, "A therapist can enhance his intervention fidelity by viewing videos of his practice sessions." Use plural pronouns instead: "Therapists can enhance their intervention fidelity by viewing videos of their practice sessions." In the 7th edition of APA, the singular use of "their" is now considered to be appropriate to refer to one person: "A therapist can enhance their intervention fidelity by viewing videos of their clinical sessions."

Race and Ethnicity

Race and ethnicity are essential in reporting standard demographics. *Race* is the classification of human groups based on specific genetic and biological markers. Race can also be based on national origin. *Ethnicity* is the classification of human groups based on cultural heritage. Race and ethnicity are based on participants' own identification, rather than the researchers'. When reporting race and ethnicity, use the preferred classification selected by participants. When constructing checklists for participants, use commonly accepted categories such as census categories and include "other" as an item with an option for participants to insert their own category. The reporting of race and ethnicity should be as specific as possible, such as Mexican American and Native American. Authors should report race and ethnicity using parallel terms, for example, African American and Asian American. Unparalleled terms in which one group is described by skin color and the other by cultural heritage (e.g., White and Pacific Islander) should be avoided. Racial and ethnic groups are considered to be proper nouns and should be capitalized: Black, White, and Alaskan American.

Disability

When writing about participants with disability, it is important to use person-first language. Person-first language is a writing style in which the participant is not defined by the presence of disability. *Participants with schizophrenia* is an example of person-first writing. Conversely, *schizophrenic participants* inappropriately characterizes the participants by the presence of schizophrenia. The exception to this rule occurs when a specific group wishes to be designated by their diagnosis, such as autism.

Similarly, language that qualifies the participants' experience through the researcher's lens is inappropriate. For example, *stroke victim*, *brain-damaged participants*, and "the participants suffered from multiple sclerosis" are examples in which the author has negatively labeled the participants' experience of disability.

The use of the word *normal* as a comparison to groups with disability is inappropriate. For example, it is inappropriate to use the following: "the normal control group," ". . . people with spinal cord injury compared to normal people in the population." The word *normal* when used to compare groups with and without disabilities implies that people having disabilities are abnormal or inferior to those without disabilities. Instead of *normal*, use *healthy control group*, *typically developed population*, and *typically developing children*.

Age

Participant ages and age ranges should always be provided as specifically as possible. Large, open-ended ranges such as *over 65* and *under 18* should be avoided. *Adolescents* refers to the age group 13–17 years, *preadolescents* refers 11–12 years, *children* refers to 1–10 years, and *infants* refers to newborns to 11-month-olds. People 18 years and older should be referred to as *adults*. The term *older adults* is preferred to the terms *seniors* and *elderly* (American Psychological Association, 2020).

Participants vs. Subjects

Traditionally the term *subjects* has been used in scientific journal writing in the hard sciences and in a time period before institutional review boards began to rigorously protect human participant and animal rights. In health care research, the term *participants* should be used instead of *subjects*. The term *subjects* implies that people may or may not know they are in a study and are being acted upon by the researcher. In health care writing, the term *participants* implies that people know they are part of a study and are actively participating.

Submission Process

Most journals have online submission systems with specific instructions and fields that must be completed to successfully submit manuscripts. Prior to submission, authors must have formatted their manuscript in full accordance with the journal's author guidelines or the paper will likely be returned. Nonadherence to page length, abstract length, table/figure count, and masking instructions are common reasons why manuscripts are returned to authors.

Most journals require authors to confirm that the manuscript is original and is not being simultaneously submitted to another journal. While online submission systems commonly require the uploading of masked manuscripts, the system will ask that corresponding author and coauthor information (e.g., names, credentials, affiliations, and email addresses) be inserted in designated fields. It is important that such information be accurate and complete because this information commonly serves as the means through which editors and journal staff contact authors. If the corresponding author's contact information changes during the manuscript review process, it is essential to notify the editor and journal staff in writing immediately.

Many journals ask that authors either submit their own similar and derivative publications or notify editors of the existence of such work to prevent inadvertent copyright issues. Electronic plagiarism check software programs are commonly used by journals to identify possible copyright problems.

Journal online submission systems commonly allow authors to recommend specific reviewers whose expertise matches the manuscript subject matter. Similarly, journals often allow authors to identify reviewers who may be inappropriate for manuscript review because of conflicting interests.

Author guidelines usually provide parameters for manuscript review length. Online systems commonly have tracking systems through which authors can monitor the status of their manuscript review. It is not appropriate to contact the editor about manuscript review status until approximately 1 month after the review time period has expired. Reviewers frequently experience unanticipated life events that may delay the submission of paper reviews. Reviewers recommended by authors may have been difficult to secure, and the review process may have been delayed. Occasionally, reviewers diverge in their recommendations, and an arbitrating reviewer must be secured who can provide a third opinion. The process of arbitration will extend the review process but will enhance its trustworthiness. If at any time during the submission and review process authors wish to withdraw their manuscript from consideration, they should contact the editor or journal staff immediately.

Checklist for Submission

- ☐ The corresponding author is identified, and contact information is provided (usually through the online system and not the manuscript).
- ☐ All coauthor information, including authorship order, has been accurately provided through the online system.
- ☐ The manuscript is fully masked.
- ☐ The manuscript formatting is congruent with the journal's designated style guidelines.
- ☐ All specific formatting guidelines that are unique to the journal and supersede the designated style guidelines have been adhered to.
- ☐ All citations in the text are referenced.
- ☐ All citations and references are congruent with regard to spelling and date.
- ☐ All tables and figures are referred to in the text and labeled in accordance with text order.
- ☐ All tables and figures have titles.

- ☐ All permissions to reprint copyrighted material have been submitted.
- ☐ Supplemental materials that may be published online, but not in hard copy, are identified and submitted.

Responding to Reviewer Recommendations

If you are invited to make revisions and resubmit your manuscript, congratulate yourself and thoroughly read all recommendations from the editor and reviewers. An invitation to revise and resubmit does not guarantee acceptance; it is important to understand requested recommendations, address revisions thoroughly, and submit a polished, higher-quality revised manuscript. The editor will likely specify instructions for responding to reviewer recommendations, but commonly authors should create a document in which all reviewer comments are listed and answered in writing. All responses to reviewer recommendations should be made in complete sentences and precisely describe how revisions address noted concerns. It is important to understand that this document will be read by both the original reviewers and editor to understand whether and how well the authors addressed noted concerns.

Responses to reviewer recommendations should be thorough and precise, as in the following examples:

> Reviewer recommendation: In the Method section, please insert a section, Interveners, in which you identify who provided intervention (type of professional), how many therapists provided intervention, their training for intervention administration, and whether interveners were anonymized to group assignment.

Answer: In the Methods section, we inserted a section labeled "Interveners" and provided the following text on p. 11: "Two occupational therapists participated in intervention administration. Both possessed over 10 years of pediatric practice experience and were trained in intervention delivery by the first author. Training consisted of a 2-day seminar presented by the first and second authors. Both interveners were anonymized to participant group assignment."

The following answers are inappropriate and do not provide sufficient information to help the reviewers and editor understand whether and how well the concern was addressed:

Answer: Done.
Answer: We added the information as requested.
Answer: This information can now be found on p. 11.

If authors do not agree with a particular reviewer recommendation, it is appropriate to write a response explaining why the revision was not needed. For example:

> Reviewer recommendation: It would be helpful to discuss the work of Strauss in the literature review and relate it to the need for your study.

Answer: We appreciate the recommendation to address Strauss' work in our literature review; however, because Strauss' work specifically addresses hemiplegia and our intervention addresses anosognosia, and because of page limitations, we decided to forgo this recommendation. Instead, we briefly discussed how Strauss' findings support our own in the Discussion section.

Most reviews are written professionally and offer constructive guidance to authors. Occasionally, reviewers inappropriately allow their emotions to permeate the language of a written review. As a result, the review language may be harsh or negative. When this occurs, authors should not personalize the tone of the review but instead focus only on the recommendations and maintain professional, neutral language in their written responses to the reviewers and editor. Maintaining professionalism includes thanking the editor and reviewers for their feedback and the opportunity to revise the manuscript.

Similarly, journal reviewers should thank authors for the opportunity to review their manuscript and adopt positive, emotionally neutral language in written reviews. All reviews should be written constructively and help authors understand how to strengthen their manuscripts. Even reviews that recommend rejection should be written positively and help authors understand how their study could be enhanced if conducted in the future.

Once authors have made requested revisions and created their "response to reviewer comments" document, the manuscript can then be resubmitted in accordance with journal guidelines. Editors commonly provide resubmission deadlines, which should be adhered to as closely as possible. If authors cannot resubmit their manuscript by a specified deadline, the corresponding author should contact the editor to request an extension. Once resubmitted, the revised manuscript will likely be reviewed by one or both of the original reviewers to determine whether the manuscript now meets publication standards. Further revisions may be requested. The manuscript revision and resubmission process is a lengthy one but provides the opportunity for authors to enhance their writing skills and become concise, precise writers.

Revising and Submitting to Another Journal if Rejected

If you receive a rejection letter from a journal, do not become discouraged. Go to the next journal on your list and determine whether that journal's publication goals match your work. Remember that journals are only able to publish a limited amount of articles, have specific publication goals, and may only publish articles about a limited topic range. Approximately 50% of rejected manuscripts are not well suited to the journal to which they were submitted. Make sure that your work matches well with the next journal to which you submit.

Go through the editor's and reviewers' comments to understand why your paper was rejected from the first journal. Make a list of noted concerns and address these as thoroughly as possible in the manuscript's next revision. Ask a neutral colleague to read your revised manuscript and provide feedback. Obtain the author guidelines from your next selected journal and reformat your manuscript to match the specified style guidelines.

The submission and publication process is lengthy and involves multiple drafts, revisions, and possible rejections (see Figure 13.1). Understanding this process, learning how to refrain from personalizing feedback and rejection, and making the time commitment for writing will help you to hurdle setbacks and rejections and persevere to eventual publication. The more frequently you go through this process, the easier it becomes.

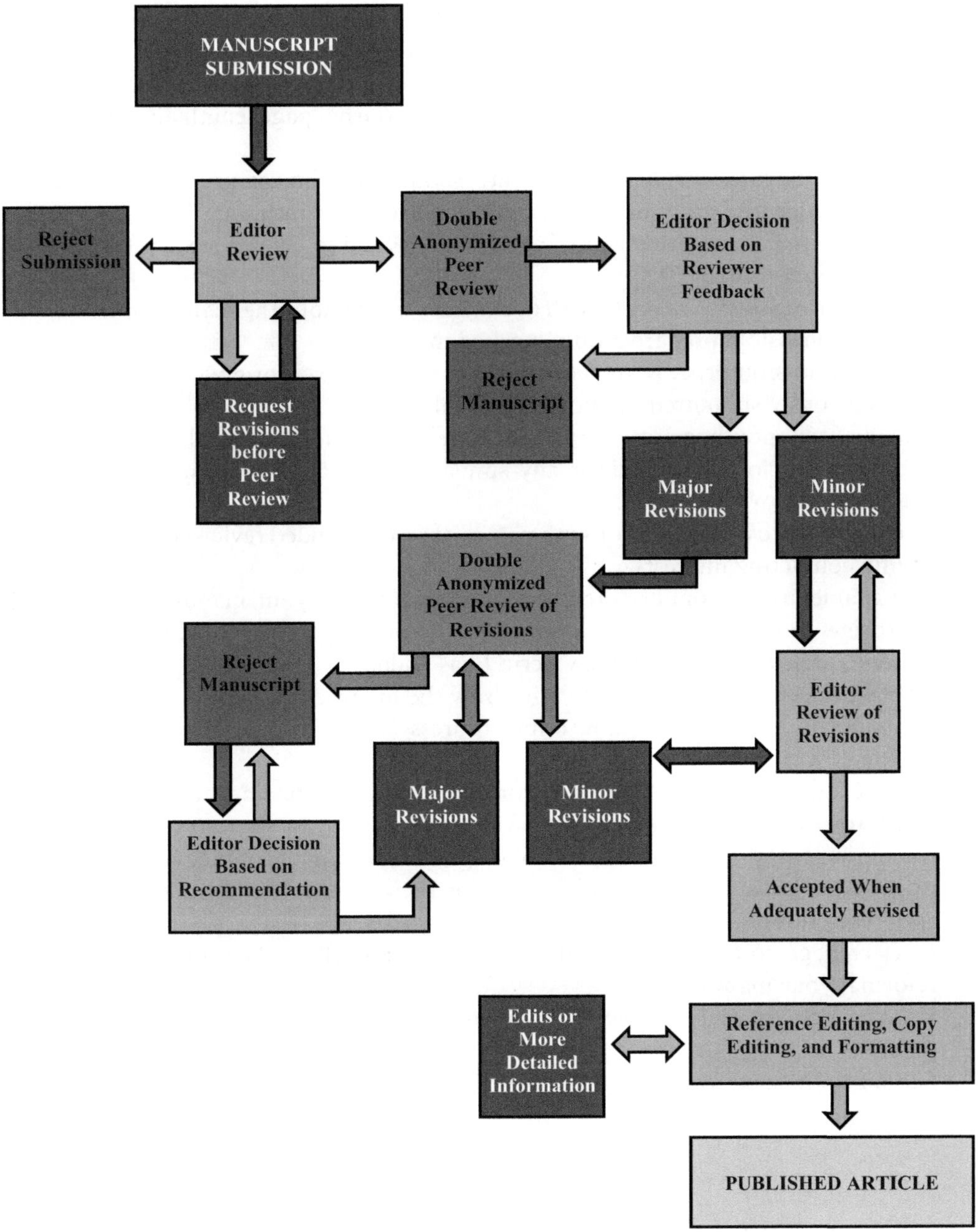

Figure 13.1 The Publication Process.

Checklist for Preparing and Submitting Manuscripts for Publication

☐ Before submission, establish author order and designate the corresponding author.

☐ Select two to three journals whose publication goals match your study or paper topic.

☐ Obtain the author guidelines of each journal to determine publication goals.

- ☐ Rank the order of journals in accordance with congruence with your work.
- ☐ Select one journal and follow that journal's style guidelines and formatting instructions.
- ☐ Make sure that the manuscript does not exceed journal page length and word count requirements.
- ☐ Work with a professional editor or neutral colleague who can proof the manuscript for concise, precise grammatical structure and sentence meaning.
- ☐ Make sure that the writing is not biased with regard to gender, sex, race and ethnicity, disability, and age.
- ☐ Use the term *participants* rather than *subjects* throughout the manuscript.
- ☐ Before submission, prepare a fully masked manuscript.
- ☐ In the submission process, indicate that the manuscript is original and is not being simultaneously submitted to another journal.
- ☐ Provide corresponding author and coauthor information fully and accurately.
- ☐ Submit or disclose to the editor any similar or derivative publications to prevent inadvertent copyright issues.
- ☐ If requested, provide the editor with names of recommended reviewers and reviewers having conflicting interests.
- ☐ If available, use the online tracking system to monitor your manuscript's status in the review process. Contact the editor only if you have not received information by 1 month after the allotted review period has ended.
- ☐ Contact the editor if you wish to withdraw the manuscript from review.
- ☐ If invited to revise your manuscript, address all editor and reviewer comments thoroughly.
- ☐ Prepare a document in which all editor and reviewer comments are listed, followed by thorough and precise answers.
- ☐ Maintain neutral and professional language and tone in all contact with editors and reviewers. Thank reviewers and editors for their feedback and the opportunity to revise and resubmit.
- ☐ If rejected, go to the next journal on your list and follow the author guidelines to reformat your manuscript.
- ☐ Use the first journal's reviewer comments to revise the manuscript as much as possible.
- ☐ Submit to the next journal.

References

American Psychological Association. (2020). *Publication manual of the American Psychological Association* (7th ed.). Author.

Conron, K. J., Mimiaga, M. J., & Landers, S. J. (2010). A population-based study of sexual orientation identity and gender differences in adult health. *American Journal of Public Health, 100(10)*, 1953–1960. doi:10.2105/AJPH.2009.174169

Rothenberg, P. S. (2013). *Race, class, and gender in the United States: An integrated study* (9th ed.). Worth.

CHAPTER 14

Writing Manuscript Cover Letters

Cover letters are often the first point of contact with the editor of a journal and therefore afford the writer the opportunity to make a good impression. Cover letters, like all scholarly writing, should be clear, concise, and accurate. Cover letters should be polite and unassuming. Manuscripts will be reviewed or not at the discretion of the editor-in-chief, and the authors should not assume that the manuscript will be sent out for review or accepted but rather take the position of requesting that the manuscript be considered for review or re-review.

There are two types of cover letters outlined in this chapter: initial submission cover letters and resubmission cover letters. Both types of cover letters should be addressed, by name, specifically to the editor-in-chief of the journal to which you are submitting. Do not address the cover letter "To Whom It May Concern." It concerns the editor-in-chief specifically. If possible, use the letterhead of the institution with which the lead author is affiliated and include the date of submission at the top.

The content of both types of cover letters should include an accurate title of the manuscript that is being submitted and a concise description of the contents of the manuscript. The authors should also discuss how the manuscript matches the mission of the journal to which they are submitting and contributes to the professional or general body of knowledge. Both types of cover letters should include a statement that makes it clear to the editors that the manuscript is being submitted exclusively to that journal by name. It is not required, but authors also may want to indicate the category of submission (e.g., Applied Research, Topics in Education, Guidelines for Practice) to ensure that no errors have been made in the submission process. Any specific disclosure statements required by the journal (e.g., use of artificial intelligence, conflicts of interest) should also be included in both cover letters. Finally, the letter should end with the credentials, contact information, and affiliations of each of the authors, with the corresponding author indicated.

In addition to the aforementioned content, the content of cover letters for resubmissions should include an acknowledgement of the feedback and a description of the revisions. Cover letters for resubmissions should thank the editor and the reviewers

DOI: 10.4324/9781003734550-14

for their feedback regarding the manuscript. The feedback is intended to strengthen the manuscript, and authors should adopt an attitude of collegiality when considering the suggestions from the editors and the reviewers. Next, a discussion of the revisions that were or were not made should be detailed. Each suggestion should be addressed with an explanation of the revision that was made or the rationale for why such a change was not warranted. If there were several suggestions, a table that addresses each suggestion individually makes it easy for the editor to understand the revisions that were made.

Checklists for Cover Letters

Initial Submission Cover Letter Checklist

- ☐ Address the cover letter to the editor-in-chief of that journal by name.
- ☐ State the title of the manuscript.
- ☐ Specify the category of submission.
- ☐ Ask for the manuscript to be considered for review for potential publication in that specific journal.
- ☐ Indicate how the content of the manuscript matches the mission of the journal.
- ☐ Discuss the contribution the manuscript makes to the profession or body of knowledge in general.
- ☐ Include a statement of exclusive submission to the journal, specifically by the journal name.
- ☐ Complete any disclosure statements that are required by the journal.
- ☐ End with the credentials, contact information, and affiliations of all authors.
- ☐ Indicate the corresponding author.

Writing Exercises: Initial Cover Letters

- Identify the Editor-in-Chief of the journal to which you are submitting your manuscript.
- What is the mission statement of the journal?
- Write a "so what" statement that explains why your research would be of interest to the readers of this journal based on the mission statement and the contents of your manuscript.

Resubmission Cover Letter Checklist

- ☐ Address the cover letter to the editor-in-chief of that journal by name.
- ☐ Thank the editors and reviewers for their feedback.
- ☐ State the title and professional contribution of the manuscript.
- ☐ Indicate that this is a resubmission or a second resubmission as appropriate.
- ☐ Specify the category of submission, as sometimes the editor suggests that this should be changed.

- ☐ Restate that this is an exclusive submission to the journal, specifically by the journal name.
- ☐ Provide a detailed description of the revisions that were made in response to the feedback.
- ☐ Include a table of the comments and responses if needed to help organize this material.
- ☐ Complete any disclosure statements that are required by the journal.
- ☐ End with the credentials, contact information, and affiliations of all authors.
- ☐ Indicate the corresponding author.

Writing Exercises: Revision Cover Letters

- Make a list of all the changes that were suggested.
- Identify the changes that were made or justify why each change was not warranted.
- Create a table of the suggested changes and revisions to attach to the cover letter.
- Write a summary paragraph that explains the revisions.

Examples of Well-Written Cover Letters

Example Initial Submission Cover Letter

May 8, 2025

Dear Dr. Dirette,

I am writing to submit my manuscript titled, "A Comprehensive Vision Screen Toolkit for Occupational Therapists within the Inpatient Rehab Setting for Patients Post Brain Injury: A Feasibility Study" for consideration as an applied research article within the *Open Journal of Occupational Therapy*. This qualitative study utilizes a thematic analysis design via semi-structured focus groups to examine the feasibility and acceptability of a new vision screen toolkit by discussing the current practices amongst occupational therapists in the inpatient rehab setting, presenting participants with education on the elements of the new screen, and gathering feedback following their personal review of it. Our findings aim to confirm that this is a tool that is highly needed and desired within this practice setting and one that therapists will find useful within their evaluation process.

Given that in prior research, occupational therapists have identified several barriers to completing vision screens, with some of the key limitations being a lack of resources, a lack of education/training, and a lack of time, we believe that the findings presented in our paper will appeal to the practicing therapists who subscribe to the *Open Journal of Occupational Therapy*. Our findings will further identify a current gap in care and address the need for a comprehensive vision screen tool that takes into consideration the unique needs of inpatient rehab settings and those patients they serve within the setting.

This manuscript examines a common issue within the realm of vision care and occupational therapy. However, it is conducted within a different practice setting than those explored in the following papers, also published by the *Open Journal of Occupational Therapy*.

1. "*Concussion-related Vision Disorder Practice Patterns in Occupational Therapy: A Survey*" by Reiser et al. (2020)
2. "*An Occupation-Based Approach to Management of Concussion: Guidelines for Practice*" by Finn (2019)

The authors confirm that this manuscript has not been previously published and is not currently under consideration by any other journal. Additionally, all of the authors have approved the contents of this paper and have agreed to the *Open Journal of Occupational Therapy's* submission policies.

Each named author has substantially contributed to conducting the underlying research and drafting this manuscript. Additionally, to the best of our knowledge, the named authors have no conflict of interest, financial or otherwise.

Sincerely,
Charisa Smith OTD, OTR/L, CBIS, Remedial Vision Specialist
Kristen Keech OTD, OTR/L CBIST
Sharon G. Wagener OTD, OTR/L

Example Resubmission Cover Letter

September 8, 2025

Dear Dr. Dirette and the *OJOT* Editorial Team:

We are pleased to resubmit our manuscript (#2536) titled **"Deliberate Practice in Occupational Therapy Education: A Conceptual Model for Professional Growth"** for consideration for publication in the *Open Journal of Occupational Therapy (OJOT)*. This paper presents a conceptual model using a scholarship of integration approach and outlines related guiding principles for occupational therapy educators that support inclusive and supportive educational practices. Through the incorporation of your feedback, we have now strengthened our argument as to why the Model for Deliberate OT Practice (MDOTP), as a contemporary, conceptual model, is a valuable addition in occupational therapy education at this point in time. We have also expanded on the implications for occupational therapy practice, especially for occupational therapy assistant and occupational therapy doctorate program utilization. Please see the chart below that outlines reviewer comments and the author's responses.

Thank you for your continued consideration.

Reviewer Comments	**Author Revisions**
Consider the unique perspective you are adding to the body of theoretical literature. Consider why this model is needed at this time in OT education. Strengthen the justification to include why, rather than just what it is.	• Justification for introducing a contemporary conceptual model considering healthcare and societal needs is included under the "Introduction" section. • Authors have added explanatory paragraphs under the section "Model for Deliberate OT Practice" that justify why this model is needed at this time in OT education.
Is this only for occupational therapists, or could the model fit into OTA education? Clarity here would help.	• This model could be applied to occupational therapy assistant education as well as entry-level OTD programs. Authors added clarification for implications under "Implications for OT Education."
Check APA use: In-text citations should be in alphabetical order. The OTPF-4 is not cited correctly. Reference page: check use of capitalization, and no city is needed in book references.	• In-text citations placed in alphabetical order • OTPF-4 citation now correctly cited • Review and revision of reference list for APA 7th edition compliance
Consider the peer reviewer feedback.	• Authors added an outer border on Figure 1 that includes Context, Environment, and Community. This relays that TUS, FoK, and SLB* realities are happening within these constructs. • Authors received, reviewed, and incorporated reviewer feedback. Thank you!

*Therapeutic Use of Self (TUS), Funds of Knowledge (FoK), Street-Level Bureaucracy (SLB).

Sincerely,

Suzanne Marasco, EdD, MS, OTR/L
Matthew Witenstein, PhD

CHAPTER 15

The Revision Process

The process of writing and submitting a paper to a scholarly journal involves revision in which reviewers and editors provide feedback and recommendations to enhance a manuscript's publication readiness. All manuscripts—even those written by seasoned scholars—go through the revision process. As authors, we may have already revised papers through multiple drafts before submission. Revisions requested by journal reviewers and editors may feel extraneous after revisions that authors have made prior to submission. However, journal reviewer recommendations are important because they emerge through the lens of professionals who best understand the publication requirements and objectives of a particular journal to which the paper was submitted.

As authors we may become attached to our writing and feel resistant to revision requests. Such attachment often hinders our ability to understand how papers can be improved. It is important to remember that all published articles have gone through moderate to extensive revisions after initial journal submission. Even after paper acceptance, copyeditors will likely further edit papers to enhance clarity and reduce word length. These steps are important components of the revision process and, while difficult to experience emotionally, ultimately enhance an article's final presentation.

Depersonalizing Reviewer Feedback

Reviewer feedback can feel critical even when it was not intended to be. It is important to set aside emotions when receiving reviewer feedback to best understand how requested revisions can strengthen a manuscript. To depersonalize reviewer comments, it is important that authors view their paper as a draft that will be revised and strengthened multiple times. After initially reading reviewer feedback, it is often beneficial to set the manuscript aside for a day or more before making revisions. This time may help authors to reduce initial emotional reactions to reviewer feedback and begin to perceive how requested revisions can be incorporated.

DOI: 10.4324/9781003734550-15

Occasionally, reviewer comments can be harsh and unprofessional. Reviews should not be written in emotionally laden language or negative comments. Editors are responsible for flagging unprofessionally written reviews and addressing them before they are provided to authors. Unfortunately, unprofessionally written reviews are not always modified before reaching authors. When authors receive such reviews, they must separate themselves emotionally from the review language and concentrate on the feedback that can be used to strengthen their manuscript.

It is important that authors do not become so daunted by reviewer feedback that they postpone making revisions and allow a paper to die. Publication requires perseverance and a thick skin able to withstand critique. The more authors experience the journal writing and submission process, the easier it becomes.

Understanding Review Feedback

After separating authors' emotions from the review process—so that emotions do not influence the ability to understand reviewer feedback—authors should reread all comments and begin to generate ideas for incorporating requested revisions into the next draft. It is important at this stage that authors fully understand what reviewers have requested. If authors are uncertain regarding the meaning of reviewer feedback for a specific item, they should first consult with coauthors and colleagues. The editor should be contacted directly if a specific reviewer comment cannot be interpreted.

Once they understand all comments, authors should identify those revisions that will be addressed and generate ideas about how revisions will be made. Occasionally, reviewers request revisions that authors believe to be inappropriate. It is suitable for authors to refrain from making a specific requested revision when such a revision may move the paper in an unintended direction or add significant word length that is incongruent with journal guidelines. In this case, authors should justify their decision in writing to the editor and reviewers (as discussed later in this chapter).

Editors often specify due dates by which revisions should be resubmitted, and such due dates should be adhered to as closely as possible. When authors cannot resubmit by a specific due date, they should request a written extension from the editor. Certain types of revisions will require greater time and effort than others. For example, updating references, reducing word count, and adding minor detail are revisions that can be made relatively quickly. Most papers require reducing detail in the Introduction section, inserting additional clarifying information in the Method section, and elaborating on interpretive information provided in the Discussion section. These types of revisions require greater time and labor. Revisions requiring statistical reanalysis, reorganization of content, substantial addition of information, and reinterpretation of results are the most labor intensive and require a comprehensive overhaul. It is essential to correctly estimate the time needed for revisions, develop a timeline, and adhere to it so that the manuscript can be resubmitted by the appointed due date. Manuscripts that are not resubmitted by the appointed due date and have not received an extension from the editor will often be withdrawn by a journal.

Adhering to Word Limits

During the revision process, it is critical to adhere to the journal's specified word and page counts. Many authors who are asked to insert background, clarifying, and interpretative information make the mistake of adding content without adjusting other manuscript sections to adhere to the journal's word limit. Revisions that exceed the maximum length by several hundred words are often resubmitted without thought to word count specifications. This oversight prolongs the revision process because the paper must be revised again to reduce word count. Before authors begin revisions, they should recheck journal guidelines regarding word count and reread the editor's cover letter to determine whether they must maintain this limit or are permitted to exceed it by a circumscribed amount. If in doubt, authors should contact the editor about word count limitations.

Responding to Reviewer Comments

Editors commonly provide instructions to authors indicating how responses to reviewer comments should be made. In addition to making requested revisions directly in the manuscript text, most journals request that authors generate a separate document in which they list all reviewer comments followed by author responses. Editors and reviewers will consult this document to understand how authors addressed each requested revision item. Authors should not take a casual approach to making these responses. All author responses should be made in complete, clear sentences that directly answer reviewer questions and concerns.

Example of Appropriate Response to Reviewers

Reviewer comment: In the Data Analysis section of the Methods, please specify which statistical test was used to determine whether differences between treatment and control groups existed at baseline. Please provide a citation for this test.

Author response: In the Data Analysis section of the Methods, we inserted the following sentence: "A Wilcoxon signed-rank test was used to determine whether a statistically significant difference existed between treatment and control groups on pretest scores (Watkins, 2020)."

Example of Inappropriate Responses to Reviewers

Author response: Done.
Author response: We added this information.
Author response: This information is now added at line 113.

Justifying Omission of Requested Revisions

Occasionally, reviewers request revisions that are incongruent with the authors' study objectives and intent. Authors do not need to make all requested revisions if they are able to justify why a specific requested revision is unsuitable. Such justifications should be made in the document listing responses to reviewer comments.

Example

Reviewer comment: Please include information about transactional theory in the introduction and relate this information to the theoretical basis for your intervention.

Author response: Thank you for this suggestion. Although we agree that transactional theory could be viewed as a basis for our intervention, we did not use this theory in our intervention development process. As noted in the Introduction, we instead used Prochaska and DiClemente's stages of change model (transtheoretical theory) as a basis for our intervention. Because of manuscript length limitations and because of additional requested content that further added page length, we chose not to address an additional theoretical base in the Introduction. We will, however, defer to the editor regarding this decision.

In the previous author response, the authors address the recommendation by thanking the reviewer for the suggestion and using appropriate language to explain why an additional theoretical base would be redundant. The authors do not suggest that the recommendation is unsuitable. Rather, they use neutral language to explain that an additional theory description would add word length that would cause the paper to exceed specified limitations. They appropriately end their response by stating that they will make this revision if desired by the editor.

Although reviewer recommendations can be challenged by authors, authors should generally comply with editor instructions—particularly when instructions address such things as word count length, formatting requirements, style guide use, heading use, and compliance with standard research reporting guidelines. Failure to defer to the above types of editor directions can result in paper rejection. Authors should not petition editors for permission to extend manuscript page length or table and figure counts.

Etiquette of the Review Process

The review process has its own set of etiquette rules that govern author, editor, and reviewer roles and behaviors. All parties should maintain neutral, positive language in all correspondence. Before the advent of email, when journal correspondence was carried out through mailed letters, correspondence adhered to widely accepted rules for professional behavior and language. Email and the breakdown of our society's social formality have loosened rules for journal correspondence. Too often, the instantaneous communication of email has encouraged people to send inappropriate, unprofessional correspondence in immediate reaction, without thinking about consequences. We urge authors to send well-considered correspondence after sufficiently processing emotional reactions in response to the review process. We also recommend the following guidelines for correspondence:

- Authors should not send correspondence when they have an emotional response to the review process. It is beneficial to wait several days to process emotions before sending correspondence.
- All correspondence should use positive language. Even if authors believe that they received an unprofessional review with emotionally laden language, it is essential not to respond similarly.

- All language in the document listing responses to reviewer comments should be neutral and positive, even if authors believe that the reviewer was unprofessional.
- To maintain professionalism, authors should thank the editor and reviewers for their help in all correspondence, particularly in their responses to reviewer comments.
- Authors should use the journal's online tracking system to determine the status of their manuscript review. Authors should not contact the editor until 1 month has expired beyond the allotted review time. A journal's author guidelines will usually specify the average review length; however, reviewer crises and difficulty securing appropriate reviewers for a specific topic can slow the average review process.
- Authors should not contact the journal to persuade the editor to review the manuscript faster to accommodate author needs (e.g., publications needed to apply for promotion or tenure or a desire to have articles published in the same issue).
- Authors should expect at least two manuscript revisions and resubmissions before acceptance.
- Authors should understand that manuscript revision does not guarantee acceptance. On occasion, authors are not able to make revisions in accordance with journal standards despite considerable help from editors and reviewers.

Proofread Prior to Resubmission

After requested revisions have been completed and prior to journal resubmission, authors should thoroughly proof the revised manuscript to identify and correct grammatical and stylistic errors, inconsistencies between citations and references, and inconsistencies between text and tables. Table numbers and heading levels can be mislabeled and lose organization through multiple paper drafts. Such problems commonly occur inadvertently during manuscript revisions. When unidentified and uncorrected, such errors can make a manuscript appear sloppily and hastily revised and further prolong the review process. On occasion authors become so familiar with a manuscript that they no longer easily see errors. In such cases, it is beneficial to have a coauthor or colleague proof the text before resubmission.

Example of a Manuscript Revision Process

To illustrate how a submitted manuscript is revised based on reviewer feedback, I present the initial and revised drafts of the article *Development and Psychometric Properties of the Emotional Intelligence Admission Essay Scale* (Gutman & Falk-Kessler, 2016). Reviewer comments and author responses are also included. This article was published in the 2016 summer issue of the *Open Journal of Occupational Therapy*, which is an open-access journal in which authors retain copyright. Reviewer comments are provided with permission of the journal's editor in chief. Please note that this article was published when the APA manual was in its 6th edition; however, the following formatted text has been updated to the APA 7th edition.

EMOTIONAL INTELLIGENCE ADMISSION ESSAY SCALE

Development and Psychometric Properties of the Emotional Intelligence Admission Essay Scale

Sharon A. Gutman
Janet P. Falk-Kessler

Abstract

Objective: The purpose was to describe the development and psychometric properties of the Emotional Intelligence Admission Essay scale.

Methods: The authors developed an admission essay question and rating scale designed to provide information about applicants' emotional intelligence (EI). Content validity, convergent validity, interrater reliability, and internal consistency were established. The scale was also examined to determine if it could discriminate between students with and without professional behavior problems in the academic and fieldwork settings.

Results: Content validity was found to be high by a panel of three experts in EI (content validity index = 1.0). Convergent validity with the Assessing Emotions Scale was moderate ($r = .46$, $p < .02$). Interrater reliability between two trained faculty raters was high ($ICC = .91$, $p < .000$). Internal consistency of the scale was high with a Cronbach's alpha of .95. This version of the scale was not able to discriminate between students with and without professional behavior problems. Conclusion: The moderate to strong psychometric properties suggest that the EI Admission Essay Scale has the ability to provide information about applicants' EI. The wording of the essay question must be modified to better instruct applicants to address interpersonal conflict.

Keywords: occupational therapy, admission selection, instrument development

Emotional intelligence (EI) is a form of social intelligence that involves the ability to recognize and appraise emotions in oneself and others, regulate and manage emotions in oneself and others, and use emotion-based information to guide behavior and problem solving (Arora et al., 2010). The term was first developed by Salovey and Mayer (1990) who argued that EI was a distinct set of skills that were separate from personality traits and previously identified types of intelligence. Later researchers extended the definition of EI by dissecting the construct into inter- and intrapersonal intelligences wherein interpersonal intelligence involves the ability to accurately read and assess other's verbal and nonverbal expressions; easily build rapport with others using an open, compassionate countenance that demonstrates interest in others;

and successfully diffuse and negotiate interpersonal conflict (Carrothers et al., 2000; McQueen, 2004). Intrapersonal intelligence involves the ability to recognize emotion in oneself and understand its origin, be aware of how one's emotions impact one's behaviors and influence others, and monitor and regulate one's emotions to enhance emotional stability and wellness (Elam, 2000; McQueen, 2004).

Emotional intelligence is a critical skill for occupational therapists, and clinical competencies relating to EI involve the ability to collaboratively work with a team of health care professionals; identify and manage patient emotions to adeptly address patient concerns and needs; identify and manage team member emotions to promote patient advocacy and diffuse possible professional domain conflicts; communicate with patients, family members, caregivers, health care providers, and insurers to ensure optimal patient care; educate caregivers who may feel overwhelmed and ill-prepared to assume caregiving responsibilities; and work cooperatively and compassionately with people from varied and diverse cultural groups (McQueen, 2004; Victoroff & Boyatzis, 2013). Given the great extent of clinical competencies that directly relate to emotional intelligence, it is surprising that this construct has not been formally examined in occupational therapy admission selection criteria.

Occupational therapy program admission selection criteria have traditionally relied upon the cognitive measures of cumulative grade point average (GPA), prerequisite GPA, science GPA, and preadmission standardized tests such as the Graduate Record Exam (GRE) (Romanelli et al., 2006). Traditionally used noncognitive measures have included interviews, personal statements and essays, volunteerism, and prior service and healthcare experience (Jones-Schenk & Harper, 2014). While the above cognitive and noncognitive measures have been shown to provide accurate predictive information about an applicant's academic performance in graduate school (Carr, 2009), they do not provide information about an applicant's potential clinical performance and professional behaviors in the academic program and fieldwork experiences. Given the large number of occupational therapy clinical competencies that relate to EI, it seems prudent to have an admission criterion that measures an applicant's EI and can identify students who have both the academic skill and EI needed to succeed in an occupational therapy program and career. The need for an EI measure in the admission selection process has been elevated by the growing number of occupational therapy school applications in the last decades (American Occupational Therapy Association [AOTA], 2014), the inflation of academic grades at the college and university level lessening the rigor of GPA as a reliable assessment measure (Jewell et al., 2013), and the generational difference in students applying to health care programs who may have values and professional behaviors that are incongruent with health care professions and who may be qualitatively different from applicants of past decades (Romanelli et al., 2006).

Other health care professions have begun to recognize the value of using EI measures in the admission selection process. Much of the literature addressing the EI of health care student applicants has been generated by the professions of medicine, nursing, dentistry, and pharmacy (Arora et al., 2010; Lyon et al., 2013; Romanelli et al., 2006; Victoroff & Boyatzis, 2013). These studies have found that students with high levels of EI as measured on standardized assessments demonstrate higher levels of clinical performance (Codier et al., 2015; Hannah et al., 2009; Rankin, 2013), are more highly rated by clinical supervisors and patients (Arora et al., 2010; Hannah et al., 2009; Rankin, 2013; Victoroff & Boyatzis, 2013), are more likely to complete their professional health care education programs (Jones-Schenk & Harper, 2014; Rankin, 2013), and are better able to work collaboratively on treatment teams as assessed by supervisors (Arora et al., 2010; Victoroff & Boyatzis, 2013). Most of the EI measures used in these studies were administered to students already matriculated in health care programs, and all authors supported the need for the incorporation of EI measures administered during the admission process.

Although the need for and value of EI measures used during the admission selection process of health care programs is clear, the most practical and reliable type of EI measure is of debate. The most commonly available form of EI measure is a paper and pencil or computer generated test (Arora et al., 2010). Such assessments either pose scenarios and ask respondents to identify the most emotionally intelligent answer through a multiple choice format or are self-report measures that ask respondents to identify to what extent they identify with a specific skill (e.g., "I am able to read other's facial expressions to determine their mood.") (Fiori & Antonakis, 2011). Another form of EI assessment gaining interest among health care programs is the structured interview, in which a specific set of questions is asked of all applicants (Latif, 2004; Levashina et al., 2014; Pau et al., 2013). In the structured interview, applicants may be consecutively interviewed by several interviewers who are all trained in interview administration and have established interrater reliability in the use of a standardized EI rating scale. While the use of face-to-face structured interviews and standardized paper and pencil or computer generated tests are often reliable and valid, they can be costly and labor intensive. Most EI measures with established reliability and validity are expensive and an administration fee is charged per student. Structured interviewing is time and labor intensive and requires training interviewers in both administration and assessment.

In response to the need to incorporate a practical and reliable EI measure into the admission selection process, the faculty in the Occupational Therapy Program at Columbia University Medical Center (CUMC), have developed an essay question and rating scale, the EI Admission Essay Scale, which may have the ability to provide information about an applicant's EI. The essay question asks applicants to describe a conflict situation in a work, school, or personal event; how the applicant knowingly or unknowingly contributed to the conflict; and how they attempted to resolve the conflict based on the ability to use emotion based information to guide problem solving. The instrument used to assess the applicant's essay is a 5-item, 4-point Likert scale with a range from 0 (no evidence) to 3 (strong evidence). The purpose of the present study was to develop the pilot version of the EI Admission Essay Scale and establish content and convergent validity, interrater reliability, and internal consistency. Additionally, we hoped to determine whether the scale is able to discriminate between students who have professional behavior problems in the academic and fieldwork setting and students who do not.

The research questions were:

1 Can an admission essay question and rating scale be developed to provide information about an applicant's EI?
2 Using a panel of three experts in emotional intelligence research, what is the content validity of the EI Admission Essay Scale?
3 Does the EI Admission Essay Scale have convergent validity with the Assessing Emotions Scale (Schutte et al., 1998, 2009)?
4 Using trained occupational therapy faculty raters, can interrater reliability be established for the EI Admission Essay Scale?
5 What is the internal consistency of the EI Admission Essay Scale using data from first year students in the CUMC Occupational Therapy Entry-Level Program?
6 Can the EI Admission Essay Scale discriminate between students who have professional behavior problems in the academic and/or fieldwork setting and students who do not?

Method

Research Design

This study described the development of a pilot assessment intended to measure EI in occupational therapy program applicants. Psychometric properties of the pilot instrument that were established included content and convergent validity, interrater reliability, and internal consistency as described below. We additionally examined whether the EI Admission Essay Scale could discriminate between students with and without professional behavior problems. CUMC's IRB approved this study and all participants provided consent.

Phase 1: Content Validity

Participants

To establish content validity of the EI Admission Essay Scale we assembled a panel of three professionals having expertise in EI research and literature. One expert was a physician educator who developed and implemented admission interview procedures for medical school applicants to ascertain information about EI. A second expert was a director of student wellness at a large, urban, northeastern university and specialized in emotional intelligence. A third expert was a professor in the Center for Educational Research and Evaluation at CUMC and taught coursework in EI.

Procedures

To develop the essay question and rating scale, the authors completed a literature review of emotional intelligence research and divided the construct into its component parts of intra- and interpersonal intelligence. Since successful conflict negotiation is a key determinant of higher levels of emotional intelligence, we developed a question in which applicants were asked to describe a conflict situation that occurred in a work, school, or personal situation. To gain insight into the applicant's awareness of ways in which their behavior and emotions impacted others (intrapersonal intelligence), applicants were asked to describe how they may have knowingly or unknowingly contributed to the conflict. To gain information about the applicant's ability to consider others' emotions and work collaboratively (interpersonal intelligence), we then asked applicants to describe their attempts at conflict resolution. Applicants were asked to address this question in 750 words. The question read as follows: "Describe a conflict that existed in a class, job, or life event in which you were a participant. How did you contribute wittingly or unwittingly to this conflict? How was the conflict handled by all involved parties?"

To develop a rating scale that could evaluate the EI content of the essay, we returned to our list of component parts of EI and formulated five scale items that addressed both intra- and interpersonal intelligence as described next. The scale items more heavily focus on interpersonal skills since such skills underlie a majority of clinical professional behaviors.

1 The applicant was able to place self in others' shoes to understand others' experiences, emotions, and perspectives in a conflict situation. (Interpersonal intelligence)
2 The applicant was able to understand how one's own actions contributed to a conflict. (Intrapersonal intelligence)
3 The applicant attempted to understand the conflict situation without blaming others for the conflict. (Interpersonal intelligence)
4 The applicant attempted to create a resolution that benefited all parties of a conflict to the greatest extent possible. (Interpersonal intelligence)
5 The applicant was able to cooperate equally with others in a conflict situation to problem solve and form a resolution to the conflict (i.e., did not monopolize problem solving or present oneself as hero). (Interpersonal intelligence)

Data Collection

Expert raters were then provided with the essay question, list of scale items, and a rating scale form and were asked to complete and return the rating form via email. Experts did not consult with one another or have access to each other's scores.

Data Analysis
We then completed a content validity ratio (CVR) (Lawshe, 1975) by asking the three experts to determine whether each scale item was congruent with the construct of EI. Experts rated each scale item using a three-point scale where 0 = not essential, 1 = useful, and 2 = essential. The CVR for each item was calculated using the formula below, where ne is the number of experts who rated the item as essential and N is the total number of experts.

$$\text{CVR} = \frac{\text{ne} - \text{N}/2}{\text{N}/2}$$

A content validity index (CVI), the score for the entire instrument, was then calculated by determining the mean for all retained items (Lawshe suggests that items receiving a 0 be discarded). Using a content validity index, items require a .83 level of endorsement to establish content validity (DeVon et al., 2007); however, if 4 or fewer raters are used, the CVR for each item must be 1 to demonstrate content validity.

After content validity was established for the five scale items, we developed a 4-point rating scale for all items where 0 = no evidence, 1 = minimal evidence, 2 = moderate evidence, and 3 = strong evidence. Possible total scores range from 0 to 15 with higher scores indicating higher EI.

Results
All three experts rated each of the five essay scale items as essential (2.0) which resulted in a CVR of 1.0 for each item and a CVI of 1.0 for the entire scale. As a result, this pilot version of the scale was determined to have high content validity with the construct of EI.

Phase 2: Convergent Validity

Participants
To enroll in this study participants had to be matriculated first or second year students in the CUMC Occupational Therapy Entry-Level Program who completed the EI Admission Essay Scale as part of their application process. Participation was voluntary and students could choose not to participate. Students were recruited through an email invitation with an embedded link to an online version of the Assessing Emotions Scale (Schutte et al., 1998, 2009). We retrospectively collected admission essay questions of applicants enrolled as current first and second year students.

Procedures
To establish convergent validity we correlated EI Admission Essay Scale scores of 40 first and second year students with their scores on the Assessing Emotions Scale

(Schutte et al., 1998, 2009). The Assessing Emotions Scale is a self-report measure of EI based on Salovey and Mayer's (1990) original model of EI (Mayer & Salovey, 1993). The scale has 33 items, uses a 5-point scale (1 = strongly disagree, 2 = somewhat disagree, 3 = neither agree nor disagree, 4 = somewhat agree, 5 = strongly agree), and requires approximately 5 minutes to complete. Total scores range from 33 to 165 with higher scores indicating higher levels of EI. Internal consistency of the scale was reported to be high with a Cronbach's alpha of .90 (Schutte et al., 1998, 2009). Schutte also reported that test-retest reliability was moderately high ($r = .78$, $p < .05$). Convergent validity with the Emotional Quotient Inventory (Bar-On, 1997) was found to be moderate ($r = .43$, $p < .05$) (Schutte et al., 1998, 2009).

Data Collection

Both first and second year participating students completed the Assessing Emotions Scale during the same 1-month period; however, first year students completed the scale in the first semester of their academic program, while second year students completed the scale in the third semester of their academic program. To determine that length in the academic program did not influence student EI scores, we analyzed whether a statistically significant difference existed between first and second year student scores on both the EI Admission Essay Scale and the Assessing Emotions Scale.

The essay questions, which had been completed as part of the application process, were retrieved from student files by an admissions coordinator who coded and masked them. Students completed the Assessing Emotions Scale anonymously using their university ID numbers as codes. The master list linking codes to student names was maintained electronically on a password protected and encrypted computer by the admissions coordinator.

Both authors rated all 40 student EI Admission Essay Scales, first separately and then together to establish consensus when disagreement occurred. All essays were masked and authors were anonymized to each other's initial scores. Interrater reliability between both authors was found to be high for separate, anonymized ratings ($ICC = .94$, $p < .01$).

Data Analysis

Data were entered into SPSS version 21 and level of significance was set at .05. To determine if EI Admission Essay Scale scores correlated with scores of the Assessing Emotions Scale, a Spearman rho correlation coefficient was used (Portney & Watkins, 2013).

Results

The data from 27 first year and 13 second year students (N = 40; male = 7, female = 33; White = 31, Asian = 5, African American = 2, Native American = 1, Hispanic = 1) were used to establish convergent validity between the EI Admission Essay Scale and the

Assessing Emotions Scale. Convergent validity between these two scales was found to be moderate at $r = .46$, $p < .02$. Because first and second year students completed the Assessing Emotions Scale at different times in their curricula, we used a Mann Whitney U test to examine whether first and second year students differed in their EI levels (Portney & Watkins, 2013). A difference found may have been attributed to year in program; however, no statistically significant difference was found between first and second year students on both their EI Admission Essay Scale scores and the Assessing Emotions Scale scores.

Phase 3: Interrater Reliability

Participants

To establish interrater reliability of the EI Admission Essay Scale, two faculty members of the CUMC Occupational Therapy Program volunteered to serve as raters. These faculty members responded to an email invitation sent by the first author to all 10 full-time faculty members of the CUMC Occupational Therapy Program.

Procedures

The two faculty members received one hour of training in EI Admission Essay Scale rating procedures; training was provided by the first author. After training, raters were asked to separately rate three masked essays randomly selected from the total pool of 54 essays submitted by the first year class; essays were randomly selected by authors using a table of random numbers.

Data Collection

The raters' scores for the three essays were completed separately and submitted by email one day after their training period. Raters were anonymized to each other's scores.

Data Analysis

Data were entered into SPSS version 21 and level of significance was set at .05. An intraclass correlation coefficient was used to determine interrater reliability between the two trained raters (Portney & Watkins, 2013).

Results

Interrater reliability was found to be high ($ICC = .91$, $p < .000$).

Phase 4: Internal Consistency

Participants

To determine the internal consistency of the EI Admission Essay Scale, we used the retrospectively collected admission essays of the 54 applicants admitted as current first-year students (male = 10, female = 44; White = 44, Asian = 4, African American = 4, two or more races = 3).

Procedures

The essays of the 54 matriculated first year students were retrieved by the admissions coordinator who masked and coded them. Authors had already rated all essays during the procedures used to establish convergent validity. As stated above, essays were rated by both authors, first separately while anonymized to each other's scores, and then together to address the existence of differences until consensus was reached. Achieving consensus was important to create one score for each essay item so that internal consistency could be determined. Interrater reliability between both authors for anonymized rating was high ($ICC = .94$, $p < .01$). After the essays of all 54 first year students were rated by both authors and one score was established for each item (for all essays), the item scores for all essays were compared to determine internal consistency.

Data Collection

Students completed the EI essays approximately 6 to 8 months earlier as part of their admissions application. This data set was retrospectively collected for this study by the admissions coordinator. Essays were masked and authors were anonymized to each other's scores in the initial phase of rating.

Data Analysis

Data were entered into SPSS version 21 and level of significance was set at .05. To determine if a correlation existed between scale items, a Cronbach's alpha correlation coefficient was used (Portney & Watkins, 2013).

Results

Internal consistency was found to be high with a Cronbach's alpha of .95.

Phase 5: Discrimination between Problematic and Nonproblematic Students

Participants

Data were the retrospectively collected admission essays of 54 admitted first year students.

Procedures

One objective of this study was to determine if the EI Admission Essay Scale could discriminate between students who demonstrated professional behavior problems in the academic and fieldwork environments and those who did not. We decided not to determine if EI Admission Essay Scale scores correlated with student scores on the American Occupational Therapy Association (AOTA) Fieldwork Evaluation (AOTA, 2002) because raters of the AOTA assessment had not attained interrater reliability with each other. Instead, we first identified those students who demonstrated problematic professional behaviors in the academic and fieldwork environments and then determined if a statistically significant difference existed between their EI Admission Essay Scale scores and the scores of students who did not demonstrate professional behavior problems. Students who were identified as having problematic professional behaviors in the academic setting had received professional development forms and counseling from advisors. Students identified as exhibiting problematic professional behaviors in the fieldwork setting (Level I or II) had received behavioral contracts or had been withdrawn from or failed fieldwork.

Data Collection

Data used to determine whether EI Admission Essay Scale scores could discriminate between problematic and nonproblematic students were the student EI Admission Essay Scale scores, student records of professional development forms (indicating that the student was counseled by the academic advisor as a result of problematic professional behaviors), and documentation of fieldwork behavioral contracts or withdrawal/failure. Examining whether the EI Admission Essay Scale could discriminate between students with and without professional behavior problems required that we unmask and link essays with academic and fieldwork performance information. For this reason, we completed this step as a final study activity to avoid biasing the procedures used to establish convergent validity, interrater reliability, and internal consistency.

Data Analysis

To determine if the EI Admission Essay Scale could discriminate between students who experienced professional behavior problems and those who did not, we used a Mann Whitney U test (Portney & Watkins, 2013).

Results

Five students (male = 2; female = 3) demonstrated problematic professional behavior in the academic and fieldwork settings during the first year curriculum. A Mann Whitney U test showed no statistically significant difference between the EI Admission Essay Scale scores of these 5 students and the remaining 49 of the first year class. Despite a lack of statistical significance, however, it is interesting to note that these five students all obtained scores of 0 on their EI Admission Essay Scales, indicating the lowest possible score. Other students, however, also obtained

0 scores because they either failed to answer the question or showed no evidence of EI in their essays. When examining the 54 essays as a whole we found that only 18 (33.33%) answered the question and wrote about an experience of interpersonal conflict. Sixteen (29.62%) misinterpreted the question and wrote about an internal conflict that did not involve the ability to interpret and address others' emotions; 20 (37.03%) did not answer the question and wrote about their background, achievements, and career goals. Because of the large number of students who did not adequately answer the question and received low or 0 scores, it was difficult to statistically discriminate between students who possessed professional behavior problems and those who did not.

Discussion

This study aimed to determine if an admission essay scale could be developed that could capture information about an applicant's EI. The study also sought to establish the psychometric properties of content validity, convergent validity, interrater reliability, and internal consistency for this pilot version of the EI Admission Essay Scale. Because high content validity was established with a panel of experts and moderate convergent validity was found between the EI Admission Essay Scale and the Assessing Emotions Scale, we suggest that the EI Admission Essay Scale can yield information about an applicant's EI.

Although we hoped that the EI Admission Essay Scale could discriminate between students with and without professional behavior problems, we found that this version of the essay question was not able to do so, primarily because a large number of student applicants misinterpreted the question and wrote about an internal conflict rather than an interpersonal one. Although student essays addressing internal conflicts did provide some information about EI, essay content failed to address information about interpersonal intelligence. We realize that our question must be rewritten to provide clearer instructions about required essay content, particularly addressing interpersonal conflict. Once the question is rewritten we believe that the essay will have greater potential to yield information about EI and possibly predictive validity with classroom and fieldwork professional behaviors.

The high level of interrater reliability, internal consistency, and content validity established for this pilot version suggest that the scale items are easily measured and address the construct of EI. Further refinement of the actual question has the potential to produce an admission selection measure that can help occupational therapy programs more efficiently identify students with higher levels of EI.

Although we did not examine the use of the question and scale as an interview procedure, there may be potential for the instrument to be used in this way. There is some evidence that interview procedures are able to capture applicant EI more effectively than written essays due to the interviewer's ability to redirect applicants when they do not answer the question (Latif, 2004; Levashina et al., 2014; Pau et al., 2013). In our study we found that approximately one-third of applicants misinterpreted the question. Another third chose not to address the question and instead wrote about a subject of their own choosing. In an interview situation, such applicants could be redirected by the interviewer. Structured EI interviews—in which the interviewer asks structured questions about specific scenarios to yield EI information—have been found to be more time-consuming than typical admission interviews because of the time needed to redirect applicants to address desired content (Levashina et al., 2014; Pau et al., 2013). In a high-stakes situation, such as a college interview, applicants may be more guarded and hesitant to talk about their experience of interpersonal conflict. The same may be true with the question when it is used in an essay format. In our study, two thirds of applicants wrote about situations they may have perceived as safe content for a college essay, such as experiencing an internal desire to change careers. It may be likely that students with lower levels of EI are less comfortable talking about their emotions and interpersonal conflict. Further testing of the conflict question used in a face-to-face interview may provide information about which format (essay or structured interview) yields greater information about an applicant's EI.

Limitations

One limitation of the study was the small sample size and predominance of white females as participants. Although the CUMC Occupational Therapy Program has a more diverse student population compared to the national average of occupational therapy schools (AOTA, 2014), our study sample nevertheless consisted largely of young adult white females. While our sample reflects the national average, having a more diverse sample would likely yield greater information about EI in student applicants. Although our expert panel rated the scale items as having high content validity, we only used three experts. Content validity would be stronger if repeated with 5 or more experts.

Future Research

While the initially established psychometric properties of the EI Admission Essay Scale were moderate to strong, we realize that the wording of our question must be made more specific and direct applicants to write about an interpersonal conflict. Once our question is rewritten for the subsequent scale version, it will be important to reassess psychometric properties. Future research is also needed to understand if the next scale version can discriminate between students with and without professional behavior problems in the academic and fieldwork settings. Additional research could also be undertaken to understand if the question can be used in a structured admission interview format to yield information about applicant EI.

Conclusion

This study described the development of an admission essay scale designed to yield information about applicant EI and reported the scale's initial psychometric properties. Although initially established psychometric properties of the scale were moderate to strong, the wording of the essay question must be modified to help applicants focus their writing on interpersonal conflict. Despite the need for modification of question wording, findings of this study demonstrate that the EI Admission Essay Scale has the potential to be used as an admission selection criterion that can help occupational therapy programs better identify students with higher levels of EI.

References

American Occupational Therapy Association. (2002). *Fieldwork performance evaluation for the occupational therapy student*. AOTA Press.

American Occupational Therapy Association. (2014). *Academic programs annual data report: Academic year 2013–2014*. www.aota.org//media/Corporate/Files/EducationCareers/Accredit/2013-2014-Annual-Data-Report.pdf

Arora, S., Ashrafian, H., Davis, R., Athanasiou, T., Darzi, A., & Sevdalis, N. (2010). Emotional intelligence in medicine: A systematic review through the context of the ACGME competencies. *Medical Education*, 44, 749–764. https://doi.org/10.1111/j.1365-2923.2010.03709.x

Bar-On, R. (1997). *The emotional quotient inventory (EQ-i): A test of emotional intelligence*. Multi-Health Systems.

Carr, S. E. (2009). Emotional intelligence in medical students: Does it correlate with selection measures? *Medical Education*, 43(11), 1069–1077. https://doi.org/10.1111/j.1365-2923.2009.03496.x

Carrothers, R. M., Gregory, S. W., Jr., & Gallagher, T. J. (2000). Measuring emotional intelligence of medical school applicants. *Academic Medicine*, 75(5), 456–463.

Codier, E. E., Kofoed, N. A., & Peters, J. M. (2015). Graduate-entry non-nursing students: Is emotional intelligence the difference? *Nursing Education Perspectives*, 36(1), 46–47. https://doi.org/10.5480/12-874.1

DeVon, H. A., Block, M. E., Moyle-Wright, P., Ernst, D. M., Hayden, S. J., Lazzara, D. J., ... & Kostas-Polston, E. (2007). A psychometric toolbox for testing validity and reliability. *Journal of Nursing Scholarship*, 39(2), 155–164. http://onlinelibrary.wiley.com/doi/10.1111/j.1547-5069.2007.00161.x/pdf

Elam, C. L. (2000). Use of "emotional intelligence" as one measure of medical school applicants' noncognitive characteristics. *Academic Medicine*, 75(5), 445–446. http://journals.lww.com/academicmedicine/Fulltext/2000/05000/Use_of__Emotional_Intelligence__as_One_Measure_of.11.aspx

Fiori, M., & Antonakis, J. (2011). The ability model of emotional intelligence: Searching for valid measures. *Personality and Individual Differences*, 50(3), 329–334. https://doi.org/10.1016/j.paid.2010.10.010

Hannah, A., Lim, B. T., & Ayers, K. M. (2009). Emotional intelligence and clinical interview performance of dental students. *Journal of Dental Education*, 73(9), 1107–1117. https://doi.org/10.1002/j.0022-0337.2009.73.9.tb04799.x

Jewell, R. T., McPherson, M. A., & Tieslau, M. A. (2013). Whose fault is it? Assigning blame for grade inflation in higher education. *Applied Economics*, 45(9), 1185–1200. https://doi.org/10.1080/00036846.2011.621884

Jones-Schenk, J., & Harper, M. G. (2014). Emotional intelligence: An admission criterion alternative to cumulative grade point averages for prelicensure students. *Nurse Education Today*, 34(3), 413–420. https://doi.org/10.1016/j.nedt.2013.03.018

Latif, D. A. (2004). Using the structured interview for a more reliable assessment of pharmacy student applicants. *American Journal of Pharmaceutical Education*, 68(1), 1–7. https://doi.org/10.5688/aj680121

Lawshe, C. H. (1975). A quantitative approach to content validity. *Personnel Psychology*, 28(4), 563–575. https://doi.org/10.1111/j.1744-6570.1975.tb01393.x

Levashina, J., Hartwell, C. J., Morgeson, F. P., & Campion, M. A. (2014). The structured employment interview: Narrative and quantitative review of the research literature. *Personnel Psychology*, 67(1), 241–293. https://doi.org/10.1111/peps.12052

Lyon, S. R., Trotter, F., Holt, B., Powell, E., & Roe, A. (2013). Emotional intelligence and its role in recruitment of nursing students. *Nursing Standard*, 27(40), 41–46. https://doi.org/10.7748/ns2013.06.27.40.41.e7529

Mayer, J. D., & Salovey, P. (1993). The intelligence of emotional intelligence. *Intelligence*, 17, 433–442. https://doi.org/10.1016/0160-2896(93)90010-3

McQueen, A. C. (2004). Emotional intelligence in nursing work. *Journal of Advanced Nursing*, 47(1), 101–108. https://doi.org/10.1111/j.1365-2648.2004.03069.x

Pau, A., Jeevaratnam, K., Chen, Y. S., Fall, A. A., Khoo, C., & Nadarajah, V. D. (2013). The multiple mini-interview (MMI) for student selection in health professions training: A systematic review. *Medical Teacher*, 35(12), 1027–1041. https://doi.org/10.3109/0142159X.2013.829912

Portney, L. G., & Watkins, M. P. (2013). *Foundations of clinical research: Applications to practice* (3rd ed.). Pearson, Prentice Hall.

Rankin, B. (2013). Emotional intelligence: Enhancing values-based practice and compassionate care in nursing. *Journal of Advanced Nursing*, 69(12), 2717–2725. https://doi.org/10.1111/jan.12161

Romanelli, F., Cain, J., & Smith, K. M. (2006). Emotional intelligence as a predictor of academic and/or professional success. *American Journal of Pharmaceutical Education*, 70(3). https://doi.org/10.5688/aj700369

Salovey, P., & Mayer, J. D. (1990). Emotional intelligence. *Imagination, Cognition and Personality*, 9, 185–211. https://doi.org/10.2190/DUGG-P24E-52WK-6CDG

Schutte, N. S., Malouff, J. M., & Bhullar, N. (2009). The assessing emotions scale. In Stough, C., Saklofske, D., & Parker, J. (Eds.), *The assessment of emotional intelligence* (pp. 119–135). Springer.

Schutte, N. S., Malouff, J. M., Hall, L. E., Haggerty, D. J., Cooper, J. T., Golden, C. J., & Dornheim, L. (1998). Development and validation of a measure of emotional intelligence. *Personality and Individual Differences*, 25, 167–177. https://doi.org/10.1016/S0191-8869(98)00001-4

Victoroff, K. Z., & Boyatzis, R. E. (2013). What is the relationship between emotional intelligence and dental student clinical performance? *Journal of Dental Education*, 77(4), 416–426. https://doi.org/10.1002/j.0022-0337.2013.77.4.tb05487.x

Reviewer Comments with Author Responses

Reviewer 1

Reviewer comment:

This paper provides a valuable addition to the literature and a thorough approach to establishing the validity of an instrument of measure. I am wondering about the statistical power of the findings, given the small N of 40. Usually a larger sample size is required to truly determine validity of an instrument. Please address this issue in your revision. Thank you.

Author response:

Thank you for bringing to our attention that we had not adequately addressed the issue relating to small sample size. We have revised our Limitations section as follows:

> One limitation of the study was the small sample size and predominance of white females as participants. Although the CUMC Occupational Therapy Program has a more diverse student population compared to the national average of occupational therapy schools (AOTA, 2014), our study sample nevertheless consisted largely of young adult white females. While our sample reflects the national average, having a more diverse and larger sample would likely yield greater information about EI in student applicants. A larger sample size would also enhance statistical power and rigor of results. Although our expert panel rated the scale items as having high content validity, we only used three experts. Content validity would be stronger if repeated with 5 or more experts.

Reviewer 2

Reviewer comment:

Overall this manuscript is well written and discusses an interesting topic, which is applied in a novel way to occupational therapy admission procedures. I appreciate the author's attempt to provide guidance for additional measures to be used for determination of admission into occupational therapy programs and the use of a non-academic-based criterion. Primary work on the establishment of an EI measure that is efficient, valid and reliable is useful and authors examined the psychometric properties in effective ways.

Some of the issues with this manuscript are that the concept of EI as an admission criterion needs to be further developed and supported. Although authors acknowledge EI is a skill, authors propose that it is essential applicants have high levels of EI before entering an occupational therapy program. The call for EI as an essential skill prior to beginning an occupational therapy course of study is not well supported by the literature review or author's findings.

Author response:

Thank you for helping us clarify that we have not suggested that student applicants must have high levels of EI before entering occupational therapy school. We are suggesting instead that an EI measure be used along with traditional cognitive and noncognitive measures to identify applicants with *higher* levels of EI—just as admission committees seek applicants with higher grades, more health- and occupational therapy-related experience, and greater diversity of life experience. We have added the following text to the paper in the Introduction section to address the reviewer's concerns:

> Occupational therapy is now ranked as the number ninth health care job by *US News and World Report* (2015) and applications to occupational therapy schools have more than doubled in the last decade (AOTA, 2014). Applicants who may not have the propensity for a health career but who are attracted to the job security and higher salaries that health careers provide have increasingly applied to health care schools in the last decade (Buerhaus et al., 2009). It has been the authors' experience that some students have professional behavioral problems related to emotional intelligence throughout the academic and fieldwork curricula. In the Occupational Therapy Program at Columbia University Medical Center (CUMC) we receive a high amount of applications and are only able to admit 10% of our applicant pool. Our desire to identify students with higher levels of emotional intelligence—and flag students who may not be adequately suited for an occupational therapy career—underpins our effort to develop an EI admission assessment that can be used adjunctly with traditional cognitive and noncognitive measures. Occupational therapy programs that identify students with limited emotional intelligence may prefer to help students develop EI in the occupational therapy curriculum.

Reviewer comment:

Introduction:

Authors did not adequately connect the main topic area (emotional intelligence) to the admission process. Additionally, EI is a skill and many health profession curricula include EI skills training. It was not made clear why this should be measured prior to admission and used as a selection criterion for entrance if it is something that can be taught and developed.

Authors state that the need for EI is elevated by the number of applicants, but it is not clear why the number of applicants increases the need for EI measures. Also authors make a statement about generational differences and values, but this also isn't clearly linked to the need for using EI measures in the admission process.

Author response:

As mentioned above, we have more fully addressed these points in the introduction with the following text:

> Occupational therapy program admission selection criteria have traditionally relied upon the cognitive measures of cumulative grade point average (GPA), prerequisite GPA, science GPA, and preadmission standardized tests such as the Graduate Record Exam (GRE) (Romanelli, Cain, & Smith, 2006). Traditionally used noncognitive measures have included interviews, personal statements and essays, volunteerism, and prior service and healthcare experience (Jones-Schenk & Harper, 2014). While the above cognitive and noncognitive measures have been shown to provide accurate predictive information about an applicant's academic performance in graduate school (Carr, 2009), they do not provide information about an applicant's potential clinical performance and professional behaviors in the academic program and fieldwork experiences. Given the large number of occupational therapy clinical competencies that relate to EI, it seems prudent to have an admission criterion that measures an applicant's EI and can identify students who have both the academic skill and EI needed to succeed in an occupational therapy program and career. The need for an EI measure in the admission selection process has been elevated by the growing number of occupational therapy school applications in the last decades (American Occupational Therapy Association [AOTA], 2014), the inflation of academic grades at the college and university level lessening the rigor of GPA as a reliable assessment measure (Jewell, McPherson, & Tieslau, 2013), and the generational difference in students applying to health care programs who may have values and professional behaviors that are incongruent with health care professions and who may be qualitatively different from applicants of past decades (Romanelli et al., 2006). Occupational therapy is now ranked as the number ninth health care job by *US News and World Reports* (2015), and applications to occupational therapy schools have more than doubled in the last decade (AOTA, 2014). Applicants who may not have the propensity for a health career but who are attracted to the job security and higher salaries that health careers provide, have increasingly applied to health care schools in the last decade (Buerhaus et al., 2009). It has been the authors' experience that some students have professional behavioral problems related to emotional intelligence throughout the academic and fieldwork curricula. In the Occupational Therapy Program at Columbia University Medical Center (CUMC) we receive a high amount of applications and are only able to admit 10% of our applicant pool. Our desire to identify students with higher levels of emotional intelligence—and flag students who may not be adequately suited for an occupational therapy career—underpins our effort to develop an EI admission assessment that can be used adjunctly with traditional cognitive and noncognitive measures. Occupational therapy programs that identify students with limited emotional intelligence may prefer to help students develop EI in the occupational therapy curriculum.

We have also added the following text in the introduction regarding the debate about whether EI is a fairly static personality trait or a skill that can be learned:

> Research examining EI is relatively new and debate exists regarding whether EI is a personality trait that can be shaped within a set of parameters rooted in genetics and environment, or whether EI is a skill that can be taught and learned without a ceiling for potential.
>
> *(Petrides & Furnham, 2001).*

Reviewer comment:
It appears some of the citations used in the third paragraph are from secondary sources.

Author response:
We reviewed all citations and references and all are primary sources.

Reviewer comment:
Methods:
Authors should consistently use acronyms (on p. 5 authors use "Emotional Intelligence" vs. EI that is used throughout paper).

Author response:
Thank you for helping us to catch this error. We have corrected all acronyms in the paper.

Reviewer comment:
On page 7, authors indicate that more interpersonal skills are rated because these skills underlie the majority of clinical professional behaviors. This statement should be supported with a research citation, or this concept should be explored earlier in the paper.

Author response:
Thank you for helping us to better support our arguments with published data. We have now added the following citations:
McQueen, 2004; Victoroff & Boyatzis, 2013.

Reviewer comment:
Under Phase 5: Identifying how students with demonstrated problematic professional behaviors were identified would be helpful. Also, the author indicated that withdrawing or failing FW resulted in being identified as a professional behavior problem, but withdrawals and failures are not always related to professional behaviors. Did authors review the reasons for withdrawal and failure to ensure they were professional behavior problems?

Author response:
In the original text we stated that we identified students with professional behavior problems in the academic and fieldwork settings by determining whether they had received professional development forms and counseling from advisors. Students who exhibited professional behavioral problems during fieldwork had received behavioral contracts (due to professional behavioral problems) or had failed fieldwork. All of this information was confirmed with faculty, fieldwork coordinators, and fieldwork supervisors.

"Students who were identified as having problematic professional behaviors in the academic setting had received professional development forms and counseling from advisors. Students identified as exhibiting problematic professional behaviors in the fieldwork setting (Level I or II) had received behavioral contracts or had been withdrawn from or failed fieldwork."

> In the above reviewer comment, the reviewer requests information that was provided in the original text. Sometimes reviewers overlook information. Reviewing a manuscript of 25+ pages can be overwhelming, particularly when a manuscript includes a great deal of methodological steps and analysis. Rather than become defensive, we stated that this information was provided and offer the original text.

Reviewer comment:
A table demonstrating distribution of scores on the EI scale would be helpful to understand the scoring. From the description under Phase 5 it looks like there were many low scores or scores of zero. This information would be helpful earlier in relationship to the other statistical analysis.

Author response:
Thank you for this suggestion. We have added a table of raw scores to better help readers understand the data.

Reviewer comment:
Limitations:
Convergent validity: Second-year students completed the 2 measures at 2 different time points in the program. As noted earlier, EI can develop over time, and therefore second-year student ratings may have been influenced by passage of time and exposure to clinical settings/educational materials/life experiences. This might be listed as a limitation.

Author response:
Both second- and first-year students completed the two measures. Second-year students completed the Assessing Emotions Scale at the beginning of their second-year (third semester of curriculum), while first-year students completed the Assessing Emotions Scale at the beginning of their first semester. We used a Mann-Whitney to determine that there was no statistically significant difference between their Assessing Emotions Scale, despite time of completion. The following is an excerpt from the original paper:

> Data Collection: Both first and second year participating students completed the Assessing Emotions Scale during the same 1-month period; however, first year students completed the scale in the first semester of their academic program, while second year students completed the scale in the third semester of their academic program. To determine that length in the academic program did not influence

student EI scores, we analyzed whether a statistically significant difference existed between first and second year student scores on both the EI Admission Essay Scale and the Assessing Emotions Scale.

Results: The data from 27 first year and 13 second year students (N = 40; male = 7, female = 33; White = 31, Asian = 5, African American = 2, Native American = 1, Hispanic = 1) were used to establish convergent validity between the EI Admission Essay Scale and the Assessing Emotions Scale. Convergent validity between these two scales was found to be moderate at $r = .46$, $p < .02$. Because first and second year students completed the Assessing Emotions Scale at different times in their curricula, we used a Mann Whitney U test to examine whether first and second year students differed in their EI levels (Portney & Watkins, 2013). A difference found may have been attributed to year in program; however, no statistically significant difference was found between first and second year students on both their EI Admission Essay Scale scores and the Assessing Emotions Scale scores.

The above reviewer comment was another instance of a reviewer requesting information that was provided in the original text. Again, we simply stated that this information was provided and offered sections from the original paper.

Reviewer comment:
There appears to be a lack of variance in the EI Admission Essay scores, which can impact statistical analysis. Because no descriptive statistics are provided for the distribution of scores, it is difficult for the reader to determine if this is true. But, with 1/3 of respondents receiving "0" the analysis may have been impacted. This might be listed as a limitation.

Author response:
Thank you for addressing this point. We have inserted a table of raw scores so that readers can better understand the data.

Reviewer comment:

Conclusion:
The author's last statement about using the scale in admission selection to help better identify students with higher levels of EI is not supported by the research outcomes and should be restated. Use of the essay did not yield differences between those with higher and lower EI and performance. Therefore, using EI scores during admissions to determine those with higher EI will not predict performance, and including it in the admission process is not supported.

Author response:
Thank you for helping us to better report our data. We disagree with the reviewer's statement that the scale, in its present form, cannot yield information about an applicant's

EI. The current version of the EI Admission Essay Scale is moderately correlated with the Assessing Emotions Scale indicating that it has potential to identify students with higher levels of EI. What it cannot do in its present form is discriminate between students with and without professional behavioral problems in the academic and fieldwork settings. We have revised the text in question to read as follows:

> In this reviewer comment, the reviewer asserts that the assessment cannot yield differences between students with higher and lower emotional intelligence scores. This is an instance where we simply stated that we disagreed with the reviewer and her suggestion that the scale cannot discriminate between students with higher and lower EI. We explained that the scale is in fact moderately correlated with the Assessing Emotions Scale (and can differentiate between students with higher and lower EI levels), but at this point cannot discriminate between students with and without professional behavioral problems in the academic and fieldwork settings. We modified the concluding paragraph to clarify this confusion and provided the text changes.

This study described the development of an admission essay scale designed to yield information about applicant EI and reported the scale's initial psychometric properties. Although initially established psychometric properties of the scale were moderate to strong, the wording of the essay question must be modified to help applicants focus their writing on interpersonal conflict. Despite the need for modification of question wording, findings of this study demonstrate that the EI Admission Essay Scale, once revised, has potential to be used as an admission selection criterion that can help occupational therapy programs better identify students with higher levels of EI.

Reviewer comment:

Conceptually, using an EI scale may contribute to the overall picture of an applicant, but using EI in the admissions process as if it is a static personality trait may create barriers for applicants with fewer life experiences. EI can be taught, therefore the scale might aid in identifying students with low EI who will potentially have performance issues, and supplemental education can be provided to assist them in developing the needed EI skills. Nursing literature has some examples of EI curriculum.

The argument that these skills must be present upon admission is not clear given the literature review and evidence presented in this manuscript.

Author response:

We hope that we have addressed this point in the previous section—that we are not suggesting that applicants have high levels of EI before admissions. Rather we suggest that an EI Admission Essay Scale can be used as one measure to identify stronger applicants.

Revised Draft

EMOTIONAL INTELLIGENCE ADMISSION ESSAY SCALE

Development and Psychometric Properties of the Emotional Intelligence Admission Essay Scale

Sharon A. Gutman
Janet P. Falk-Kessler

Abstract

Objective: The purpose was to describe the development and psychometric properties of the Emotional Intelligence Admission Essay scale.

Methods: The authors developed an admission essay question and rating scale designed to provide information about applicants' emotional intelligence (EI). Content validity, convergent validity, interrater reliability, and internal consistency were established. The scale was also examined to determine if it could discriminate between students with and without professional behavior problems in the academic and fieldwork settings.

Results: Content validity was found to be high by a panel of three experts in EI (content validity index = 1.0). Convergent validity with the Assessing Emotions Scale was moderate ($r = .46$, $p < .02$). Interrater reliability between two trained faculty raters was high ($ICC = .91$, $p < .000$). Internal consistency of the scale was high with a Cronbach's alpha of .95. This version of the scale was not able to discriminate between students with and without professional behavior problems.

Conclusion: The moderate to strong psychometric properties suggest that the EI Admission Essay Scale has the ability to provide information about applicants' EI. The wording of the essay question must be modified to better instruct applicants to address interpersonal conflict.

Keywords: occupational therapy, admission selection, instrument development

Emotional intelligence (EI) is a form of social intelligence that involves the ability to recognize and appraise emotions in oneself and others, regulate and manage emotions in oneself and others, and use emotion based information to guide behavior and problem solving (Arora et al., 2010). The term was first developed by Salovey and Mayer (1990) who argued that EI was a distinct set of skills that were separate from personality traits and previously identified types of intelligence.

Later researchers extended the definition of EI by dissecting the construct into inter- and intrapersonal intelligences wherein interpersonal intelligence involves the ability to accurately read and assess other's verbal and nonverbal expressions; easily build rapport with others using an open, compassionate countenance that demonstrates interest in others; and successfully diffuse and negotiate interpersonal conflict (Carrothers et al., 2000; McQueen, 2004). Intrapersonal intelligence involves the ability to recognize emotion in oneself and understand its origin, be aware of how one's emotions impact one's behaviors and influence others, and monitor and regulate one's emotions to enhance emotional stability and wellness (Elam, 2000; McQueen, 2004). Research examining EI is relatively new and debate exists regarding whether EI is a personality trait that can be shaped within a set of parameters rooted in genetics and environment, or whether EI is a skill that can be taught and learned without a ceiling for potential (Petrides & Furnham, 2001).

This sentence was added to the Introduction to address the reviewer concern that we had not clarified whether emotional intelligence is a skill that can be learned or an innate personality trait.

Emotional intelligence is a critical skill for occupational therapists and clinical competencies relating to EI involve the ability to collaboratively work with a team of health care professionals; identify and manage patient emotions to adeptly address patient concerns and needs; identify and manage team member emotions to promote patient advocacy and diffuse possible professional domain conflicts; communicate with patients, family members, caregivers, health care providers, and insurers to ensure optimal patient care; educate caregivers who may feel overwhelmed and ill-prepared to assume caregiving responsibilities; and work cooperatively and compassionately with people from varied and diverse cultural groups (McQueen, 2004; Victoroff & Boyatzis, 2013). Given the great extent of clinical competencies that directly relate to emotional intelligence, it is surprising that this construct has not been formally examined in occupational therapy admission selection criteria.

Occupational therapy program admission selection criteria have traditionally relied upon the cognitive measures of cumulative grade point average (GPA), prerequisite GPA, science GPA, and preadmission standardized tests such as the Graduate Record Exam (GRE) (Romanelli et al., 2006). Traditionally used noncognitive measures have included interviews, personal statements and essays, volunteerism, and prior service and healthcare experience (Jones-Schenk & Harper, 2014). While the above cognitive and noncognitive measures have been shown to provide accurate predictive information about an applicant's academic performance in graduate school (Carr, 2009), they do not provide information about an applicant's potential clinical performance and professional behaviors in the academic program and fieldwork experiences. Given the large number of occupational therapy clinical competencies that relate to EI, it seems prudent to have an admission criterion that measures an applicant's EI and can identify students who have both the academic skill and EI needed to succeed in an occupational therapy program and career. The need for an EI measure in the admission selection process has been elevated by the growing number of occupational therapy school applications in the last decades (American Occupational Therapy Association [AOTA], 2014), the inflation of academic grades at the college and university level lessening the rigor of GPA as a reliable assessment measure (Jewell et al., 2013), and the generational difference in students applying to health care programs who may have values and professional behaviors that are incongruent with health care professions and who may be qualitatively different from applicants of past decades (Romanelli et al., 2006). Occupational therapy is now ranked as the number ninth health care job by US News and World Reports (2015) and applications to occupational therapy schools have more than doubled in the last decade (AOTA, 2014). Applicants who may not have the propensity for a health career but who are attracted to the job security and higher salaries that health careers provide, have increasingly applied to health care schools in the last decade (Buerhaus et al., 2009). It has been the authors' experience that some students have professional behavioral problems related to emotional intelligence throughout the academic and fieldwork curricula. In the Occupational Therapy Program at Columbia University Medical Center (CUMC) we receive a high amount of applications and are only able to admit 10% of our applicant pool. Our desire to identify students with higher levels of emotional intelligence–and flag students who may not be adequately suited for an occupational therapy career– underpins our effort to develop an EI admission assessment that can be used adjunctly with traditional cognitive and noncognitive measures. Occupational therapy programs that identify students with limited emotional intelligence may prefer to help students develop EI in the occupational therapy curriculum.

These sentences were added or refined from the original text in response to the reviewer's concern that we had not adequately argued that emotional intelligence is an essential admission criterion. We specifically inserted the final sentence in this paragraph to address the reviewer's concern that some students may be able to enhance their emotional intelligence through coursework in the curriculum.

Other health care professions have begun to recognize the value of using EI measures in the admission selection process. Much of the literature addressing the EI of health care student applicants has been generated by the professions of medicine, nursing, dentistry, and pharmacy (Arora et al., 2010; Lyon et al., 2013; Victoroff & Boyatzis, 2013; Romanelli et al., 2006). These studies have found that students with high levels of EI as measured on standardized assessments demonstrate higher levels of clinical performance (Codier et al., 2015; Hannah et al., 2009; Rankin, 2013), are more highly rated by clinical supervisors and patients (Arora et al., 2010; Hannah et al., 2009; Rankin, 2013; Victoroff & Boyatzis, 2013), are more likely to complete their professional health care education programs (Jones-Schenk & Harper, 2014; Rankin, 2013), and are better able to work collaboratively on treatment teams as assessed by supervisors (Arora et al., 2010; Victoroff & Boyatzis, 2013). Most of the EI measures used in these studies were administered to students already matriculated in health care programs and all authors supported the need for the incorporation of EI measures administered during the admission process.

Although the need for and value of EI measures used during the admission selection process of health care programs is clear, the most practical and reliable type of EI measure is of debate. The most commonly available form of EI measure is a paper and pencil or computer generated test (Arora et al., 2010). Such assessments either pose scenarios and ask respondents to identify the most emotionally intelligent answer through a multiple choice format or are self-report measures that ask respondents to identify to what extent they identify with a specific skill (e.g., "I am able to read other's facial expressions to determine their mood.") (Fiori & Antonakis, 2011). Another form of EI assessment gaining interest among health care programs is the structured interview, in which a specific set of questions is asked of all applicants (Latif, 2004; Levashina et al., 2014; Pau et al., 2013). In the structured interview, applicants may be consecutively interviewed by several interviewers who are all trained in interview administration and have established interrater reliability in the use of a standardized EI rating scale. While the use of face-to-face structured interviews and standardized paper and pencil or computer generated tests are often reliable and valid, they can be costly and labor intensive. Most EI measures with established reliability and validity are expensive and an administration fee is charged per student. Structured interviewing is time and labor intensive and requires training interviewers in both administration and assessment.

A reviewer found that we had spelled out "emotional intelligence" and helped us to recheck all EI acronyms in the paper.

In response to the need to incorporate a practical and reliable EI measure into the admission selection process, the faculty in the Occupational Therapy Program at CUMC have developed an essay question and rating scale, the EI Admission Essay Scale, which may have the ability to provide information about an applicant's EI. The essay question asks applicants to describe a conflict situation in a work, school, or personal event; how the applicant knowingly or unknowingly contributed to the conflict; and how he or she attempted to resolve the conflict based on the ability to use emotion based information to guide problem solving. The instrument used to assess the applicant's essay is a 5-item, 4-point Likert scale with a range from 0 (no evidence) to 3 (strong evidence). The purpose of the present study was to develop the pilot version of the EI Admission Essay Scale, and establish content and convergent validity, interrater reliability, and internal consistency. Additionally, we hoped to determine whether the scale is able to discriminate between students who have professional behavior problems in the academic and fieldwork setting and students who do not.

The research questions were:

1 Can an admission essay question and rating scale be developed to provide information about an applicant's EI?
2 Using a panel of three experts in emotional intelligence research, what is the content validity of the EI Admission Essay Scale?
3 Does the EI Admission Essay Scale have convergent validity with the Assessing Emotions Scale (Schutte et al., 1998, 2009)?
4 Using trained occupational therapy faculty raters, can interrater reliability be established for the EI Admission Essay Scale?
5 What is the internal consistency of the EI Admission Essay Scale using data from first year students in the CUMC Occupational Therapy Entry-Level Program?
6 Can the EI Admission Essay Scale discriminate between students who have professional behavior problems in the academic and/or fieldwork setting and students who do not?

Method

Research Design

This study described the development of a pilot assessment intended to measure EI in occupational therapy program applicants. Psychometric properties of the pilot instrument that were established included content and convergent validity, interrater reliability, and internal consistency as described below. We additionally examined whether the EI Admission Essay Scale could discriminate between students with and without professional behavior problems. The CUMC IRB approved this study and all participants provided consent.

Phase 1: Content Validity

Participants

To establish content validity of the EI Admission Essay Scale we assembled a panel of three professionals having expertise in EI research and literature. One expert was a physician educator who developed and implemented admission interview procedures for medical school applicants to ascertain information about EI. A second expert was a director of student wellness at a large, urban, northeastern university and specialized in emotional intelligence. A third expert was a professor in the Center for Educational Research and Evaluation at CUMC and taught coursework in EI.

Procedures

To develop the essay question and rating scale, the authors completed a literature review of EI research and divided the construct into its component parts of intra- and interpersonal intelligence. Since successful conflict negotiation is a key determinant of higher levels of EI (McQueen, 2004; & Boyatzis, 2013), we developed a question in which applicants were asked to describe a conflict situation that occurred in a work, school, or personal situation. To gain insight into the applicant's awareness of ways in which his or her behavior and emotions impacted others (intrapersonal intelligence), applicants were asked to describe how they may have knowingly or unknowingly contributed to the conflict. To gain information about the applicant's ability to consider others' emotions and work collaboratively (interpersonal intelligence), we then asked applicants to describe their attempts at conflict resolution. Applicants were asked to address this question in 750 words. The question read as follows: "Describe a conflict that existed in a class, job, or life event in which you were a participant. How did you contribute wittingly or unwittingly to this conflict? How was the conflict handled by all involved parties?"

To develop a rating scale that could evaluate the EI content of the essay, we returned to our list of component parts of EI and formulated five scale items that addressed both intra- and interpersonal intelligence as described below. The scale items more heavily focus on interpersonal skills since such skills underlie a majority of clinical professional behaviors (McQueen, 2004; Victoroff & Boyatzis, 2013).

We added these citations to support the assertion that interpersonal skills underlie a majority of clinical professional behaviors, as requested by one reviewer.

1. The applicant was able to place self in others' shoes to understand others' experiences, emotions, and perspectives in a conflict situation. (Interpersonal intelligence)
2. The applicant was able to understand how one's own actions contributed to a conflict. (Intrapersonal intelligence)
3. The applicant attempted to understand the conflict situation without blaming others for the conflict. (Interpersonal intelligence)
4. The applicant attempted to create a resolution that benefited all parties of a conflict to the greatest extent possible. (Interpersonal intelligence)
5. The applicant was able to cooperate equally with others in a conflict situation to problem solve and form a resolution to the conflict (i.e., did not monopolize problem solving or present oneself as hero). (Interpersonal intelligence)

Data Collection

Expert raters were then provided with the essay question, list of scale items, and a rating scale form and were asked to complete and return the rating form via email. Experts did not consult with one another or have access to each other's scores.

Data Analysis

We then completed a content validity ratio (CVR) (Lawshe, 1975) by asking the three experts to determine whether each scale item was congruent with the construct of EI. Experts rated each scale item using a three-point scale where 0 = not essential, 1 = useful, and 2 = essential. The CVR for each item was calculated using the formula below where ne is the number of experts who rated the item as essential and N is the total number of experts.

$$CVR = \frac{ne - N/2}{N/2}$$

A content validity index (CVI), the score for the entire instrument, was then calculated by determining the mean for all retained items (Lawshe suggests that items receiving a 0 be discarded). Using a content validity index, items require a .83 level of endorsement to establish content validity (DeVon et al., 2007); however, if 4 or fewer raters are used, the CVR for each item must be 1 to demonstrate content validity.

After content validity was established for the five scale items, we developed a 4-point rating scale for all items where 0 = no evidence, 1 = minimal evidence, 2 = moderate evidence, and 3 = strong evidence. Possible total scores range from 0 to 15 with higher scores indicating higher EI.

Results

All three experts rated each of the five essay scale items as essential (2.0) which resulted in a CVR of 1.0 for each item and a CVI of 1.0 for the entire scale. As a result, this pilot version of the scale was determined to have high content validity with the construct of EI.

Phase 2: Convergent Validity

Participants

To enroll in this study participants had to be matriculated first or second year students in the CUMC Occupational Therapy Entry-Level Program who completed the EI Admission Essay Scale as part of their application process. Participation was voluntary and students could choose not to participate. Students were recruited through an email invitation with an embedded link to an online version of the Assessing Emotions Scale (Schutte et al., 1998, 2009). We retrospectively collected admission essay questions of applicants enrolled as current first and second year students.

Procedures

To establish convergent validity we correlated EI Admission Essay Scale scores of 40 first and second year students with their scores on the Assessing Emotions Scale (Schutte et al., 1998, 2009). The Assessing Emotions Scale is a self-report measure of EI based on Salovey and Mayer's (1990) original model of EI (Mayer & Salovey, 1993). The scale has 33 items, uses a 5-point scale (1 = strongly disagree, 2 = somewhat disagree, 3 = neither agree nor disagree, 4 = somewhat agree, 5 = strongly agree), and requires approximately 5 minutes to complete. Total scores range from 33 to 165 with higher scores indicating higher levels of EI. Internal consistency of the scale was reported to be high with a Cronbach's alpha of .90 (Schutte et al., 1998, 2009). Schutte also reported that test-retest reliability was moderately high ($r = .78$, $p < .05$). Convergent validity with the Emotional Quotient Inventory (Bar-On, 1997) was found to be moderate ($r = .43$, $p < .05$) (Schutte et al., 1998, 2009).

Data Collection

Both first and second year participating students completed the Assessing Emotions Scale during the same 1-month period; however, first year students completed the scale in the first semester of their academic program, while second year students completed the scale in the third semester of their academic program. To determine that length in the academic program did not influence student EI scores, we analyzed whether a statistically significant difference existed between first and second year student scores on both the EI Admission Essay Scale and the Assessing Emotions Scale.

The essay questions, which had been completed as part of the application process, were retrieved from student files by an admissions coordinator who coded and masked them. Students completed the Assessing Emotions Scale anonymously using their university ID numbers as codes. The master list linking codes to student names was maintained electronically on a password protected and encrypted computer by the admissions coordinator.

Both authors rated all 40 student EI Admission Essay Scales, first separately and then together to establish consensus when disagreement occurred. All essays were masked and authors were anonymized to each other's initial scores. Interrater reliability between both authors was found to be high for separate, anonymized ratings ($ICC = .94$, $p < .01$).

Data Analysis

Data were entered into SPSS version 21 and level of significance was set at .05. To determine if EI Admission Essay Scale scores correlated with scores of the Assessing Emotions Scale, a Spearman rho correlation coefficient was used (Portney & Watkins, 2013).

Results

The data from 27 first year and 13 second year students (N = 40; male = 7, female = 33; White = 31, Asian = 5, African American = 2, Native American = 1, Hispanic = 1) were used to establish convergent validity between the EI Admission Essay Scale and the Assessing Emotions Scale. Convergent validity between these two scales was found to be moderate at $r = .46$, $p < .02$. Because first and second year students completed the Assessing Emotions Scale at different times in their curricula, we used a Mann Whitney U test to examine whether first and second year students differed in their EI levels (Portney & Watkins, 2013). A difference found may have been attributed to year in program; however, no statistically significant difference was found between first and second year students on both their EI Admission Essay Scale scores and the Assessing Emotions Scale scores.

Phase 3: Interrater Reliability

Participants

To establish interrater reliability of the EI Admission Essay Scale, two faculty members of the CUMC Occupational Therapy Program volunteered to serve as raters. These faculty members responded to an email invitation sent by the first author to all 10 full-time faculty members of the CUMC Occupational Therapy Program.

Procedures

The two faculty members received one hour of training in EI Admission Essay Scale rating procedures; training was provided by the first author. After training, raters were asked to separately rate three masked essays randomly selected from the total pool of 54 essays submitted by the first year class; essays were randomly selected by authors using a table of random numbers.

Data Collection
The raters' scores for the three essays were completed separately and submitted by email one day after their training period. Raters were anonymized to each other's scores.

Data Analysis
Data were entered into SPSS version 21 and level of significance was set at .05. An intraclass correlation coefficient was used to determine interrater reliability between the two trained raters (Portney & Watkins, 2013).

Results
Interrater reliability was found to be high ($ICC = .91$, $p < .000$).

Phase 4: Internal Consistency
Participants
To determine the internal consistency of the EI Admission Essay Scale, we used the retrospectively collected admission essays of the 54 applicants admitted as current first year students (male = 10, female = 44; White = 44, Asian = 4, African American = 4, two or more races = 3).

Procedures
The essays of the 54 matriculated first year students were retrieved by the admissions coordinator who masked and coded them. Authors had already rated all essays during the procedures used to establish convergent validity. As stated above, essays were rated by both authors, first separately while anonymized to each other's scores, and then together to address the existence of differences until consensus was reached. Achieving consensus was important to create one score for each essay item so that internal consistency could be determined. Interrater reliability between both authors for anonymized rating was high ($ICC = .94$, $p < .01$). After the essays of all 54 first year students were rated by both authors and one score was established for each item (for all essays), the item scores for all essays were compared to determine internal consistency.

Data Collection
Students completed the EI essays approximately 6 to 8 months earlier as part of their admissions application. This data set was retrospectively collected for this study by

the admissions coordinator. Essays were masked and authors were anonymized to each other's scores in the initial phase of rating.

Data Analysis

Data were entered into SPSS version 21 and level of significance was set at .05. To determine if a correlation existed between scale items, a Cronbach's alpha correlation coefficient was used (Portney & Watkins, 2013).

Results

Internal consistency was found to be high with a Cronbach's alpha of .95.

Phase 5: Discrimination between Problematic and Nonproblematic Students

Participants

Data were the retrospectively collected admission essays of 54 admitted first year students.

Procedures

One objective of this study was to determine if the EI Admission Essay Scale could discriminate between students who demonstrated professional behavior problems in the academic and fieldwork environments and those who did not. We decided not to determine if EI Admission Essay Scale scores correlated with student scores on the American Occupational Therapy Association (AOTA) Fieldwork Evaluation (AOTA, 2002) because raters of the AOTA assessment had not attained interrater reliability with each other. Instead, we first identified those students who demonstrated problematic professional behaviors in the academic and fieldwork environments and then determined if a statistically significant difference existed between their EI Admission Essay Scale scores and the scores of students who did not demonstrate professional behavior problems. Students who were identified as having problematic professional behaviors in the academic setting had received professional development forms and counseling from advisors. Students identified as exhibiting problematic professional behaviors in the fieldwork setting (Level I or II) had received behavioral contracts or had been withdrawn from or failed fieldwork.

Data Collection

Data used to determine whether EI Admission Essay Scale scores could discriminate between problematic and nonproblematic students were the student EI Admission Essay Scale scores, student records of professional development forms (indicating that the student was counseled by the academic advisor as a result of problematic professional behaviors), and documentation of fieldwork behavioral contracts or withdrawal/failure. Examining whether the EI Admission Essay Scale could discriminate between students with and without professional behavior problems required that we unmask and link essays with academic and fieldwork performance information. For this reason, we completed this step as a final study activity to avoid biasing the procedures used to establish convergent validity, interrater reliability, and internal consistency.

Data Analysis

To determine if the EI Admission Essay Scale could discriminate between students who experienced professional behavior problems and those who did not, we used a Mann Whitney U test (Portney & Watkins, 2013).

Results

Five students demonstrated problematic professional behavior in the academic and fieldwork settings during the first year curriculum. A Mann Whitney U test showed no statistically significant difference between the EI Admission Essay Scale scores of these 5 students and the remaining 49 of the first-year class. Despite a lack of statistical significance, however, it is interesting to note that these five students all obtained scores of 0 on their EI Admission Essay Scales, indicating the lowest possible score. Other students, however, also obtained 0 scores because they either failed to answer the question or showed no evidence of EI in their essays. When examining the 54 essays as a whole we found that only 18 (33.33%) answered the question and wrote about an experience of interpersonal conflict. Sixteen (29.62%) misinterpreted the question and wrote about an internal conflict that did not involve the ability to interpret and address others' emotions; 20 (37.03%) did not answer the question and wrote about their background, achievements, and career goals (see Table 1). Because of the large number of students who did not adequately answer the question and received low or 0 scores, it was difficult to statistically discriminate between students who possessed professional behavior problems and those who did not.

Discussion

This study aimed to determine if an admission essay scale could be developed that could capture information about an applicant's EI. The study also sought to establish the psychometric properties of content validity, convergent validity, interrater reliability, and internal consistency for this pilot version of the EI Admission Essay Scale. Because high content validity was established with a panel of experts and moderate convergent validity was found between the EI Admission Essay Scale and the Assessing Emotions Scale, we suggest that the EI Admission Essay Scale can yield information about an applicant's EI.

Although we hoped that the EI Admission Essay Scale could discriminate between students with and without professional behavior problems, we found that this version of the essay question was not able to do so, primarily because a large number of student applicants misinterpreted the question and wrote about an internal conflict rather than an interpersonal one. Although student essays addressing internal conflicts did provide some information about EI, essay content failed to address information about interpersonal intelligence. We realize that our question must be rewritten to provide clearer instructions about required essay content, particularly addressing interpersonal conflict. Once the question is rewritten we believe that the essay will have greater potential to yield information about EI and possibly predictive validity with classroom and fieldwork professional behaviors.

The high level of interrater reliability, internal consistency, and content validity established for this pilot version suggest that the scale items are easily measured and address the construct of EI. Further refinement of the actual question has the potential to produce an admission selection measure that can help occupational therapy programs more efficiently identify students with higher levels of EI.

Although we did not examine the use of the question and scale as an interview procedure, there may be potential for the instrument to be used in this way. There is some evidence that interview procedures are able to capture applicant EI more effectively than written essays due to the interviewer's ability to redirect applicants when they do not answer the question (Latif, 2004; Levashina et al., 2014; Pau et al., 2013). In our study we found that approximately one-third of applicants misinterpreted the question. Another third chose not to address the question and instead wrote about a subject of their own choosing. In an interview situation, such applicants could be redirected by the interviewer. Structured EI interviews—in which the interviewer asks structured questions about specific scenarios to yield EI information—have been found to be more time consuming than typical admission interviews because of the time needed to redirect applicants to address desired content (Levashina et al., 2014; Pau et al., 2013). In a high-stakes situation, such as a college interview, applicants may be more guarded and hesitant to talk about their experience of interpersonal conflict. The same may be true with the question when it is used in an essay format. In our study, two thirds of applicants wrote about situations they may have perceived as safe content for a college essay, such as experiencing an internal desire to change careers. It may be likely that students with lower levels of EI are less comfortable talking about their emotions and interpersonal conflict. Further testing of the conflict question used in a face-to-face interview may provide information about which format (essay or structured interview) yields greater information about an applicant's EI.

> The Limitation section was revised to better address the study's small sample size.

Limitations

One limitation of the study was the small sample size and predominance of white females as participants. Although the CUMC Occupational Therapy Program has a more diverse student population compared to the national average of occupational therapy schools (AOTA, 2014), our study sample nevertheless consisted largely of young adult white females. While our sample reflects the national average, having a more diverse and larger sample would likely yield greater information about EI in student applicants. A larger sample size would also enhance statistical power and rigor of results. Although our expert panel rated the scale items as having high content validity, we only used three experts. Content validity would be stronger if repeated with 5 or more experts.

Future Research

While the initially established psychometric properties of the EI Admission Essay Scale were moderate to strong, we realize that the wording of our question must be made more specific and direct applicants to write about an interpersonal conflict. Once our question is rewritten for the subsequent scale version, it will be important to reassess psychometric properties. Future research is also needed to understand if the next scale version can discriminate between students with and without professional behavior problems in the academic and fieldwork settings. Additional research could also be undertaken to understand if the question can be used in a structured admission interview format to yield information about applicant EI.

Conclusion

This study described the development of an admission essay scale designed to yield information about applicant EI and reported the scale's initial psychometric properties. Although initially established psychometric properties of the scale were moderate to strong, the wording of the essay question must be modified to help applicants focus their writing on interpersonal conflict. Despite the need for modification of question wording, findings of this study demonstrate that the EI Admission Essay Scale, once revised, has potential to be used as an admission selection criterion that can help occupational therapy programs better identify students with higher levels of EI.

To address a reviewer concern, we modified the concluding paragraph to emphasize that although the current version of the instrument can identify students with higher levels of EI, problems in the essay question wording must be revised before the scale can be used as an admission instrument.

References

American Occupational Therapy Association. (2002). *Fieldwork performance evaluation for the occupational therapy student*. AOTA Press.

American Occupational Therapy Association. (2014). *Academic programs annual data report: Academic year 2013–2014*. www.aota.org//media/Corporate/Files/EducationCareers/Accredit/2013-2014-Annual-Data-Report.pdf

Arora, S., Ashrafian, H., Davis, R., Athanasiou, T., Darzi, A., & Sevdalis, N. (2010). Emotional intelligence in medicine: A systematic review through the context of the ACGME competencies. *Medical Education*, *44*, 749–764. https://doi.org/10.1111/j.1365-2923.2010.03709.x

Bar-On, R. (1997). *The emotional quotient inventory (EQ-i): A test of emotional intelligence*. Multi-Health Systems.

Buerhaus, P. I., Auerbach, D. I., & Staiger, D. O. (2009). The recent surge in nurse employment: Causes and implications. *Health Affairs*, *28*(4), w657–w668. https://doi.org/10.1377/hlthaff.28.4.w657

Carr, S. E. (2009). Emotional intelligence in medical students: Does it correlate with selection measures? *Medical Education*, *43*(11), 1069–1077. https://doi.org/10.1111/j.1365-2923.2009.03496.x

Carrothers, R. M., Gregory, S. W., Jr., & Gallagher, T. J. (2000). Measuring emotional intelligence of medical school applicants. *Academic Medicine, 75*(5), 456–463. http://journals.lww.com/academicmedicine/Fulltext/2000/05000/Measuring_Emotional_Intelligence_of_Medical_School.16.aspx

Codier, E. E., Kofoed, N. A., & Peters, J. M. (2015). Graduate-entry non-nursing students: Is emotional intelligence the difference? *Nursing Education Perspectives*, *36*(1), 46–47. https://doi.org/10.5480/12-874.1

DeVon, H. A., Block, M. E., Moyle-Wright, P., Ernst, D. M., Hayden, S. J., Lazzara, D. J., ... & Kostas-Polston, E. (2007). A psychometric toolbox for testing validity and reliability. *Journal of Nursing Scholarship*, *39*(2), 155–164. http://onlinelibrary.wiley.com/doi/10.1111/j.1547-5069.2007.00161.x/pdf

Elam, C. L. (2000). Use of emotional intelligence as one measure of medical school applicants' noncognitive characteristics. *Academic Medicine*, *75*(5), 445–446. http://journals.lww.com/academicmedicine/Fulltext/2000/05000/Use_of__Emotional_Intelligence__as_One_Measure_of.11.aspx

Fiori, M., & Antonakis, J. (2011). The ability model of emotional intelligence: Searching for valid measures. *Personality and Individual Differences*, *50*(3), 329–334. https://doi.org/10.1016/j.paid.2010.10.010

Hannah, A., Lim, B. T., & Ayers, K. M. (2009). Emotional intelligence and clinical interview performance of dental students. *Journal of Dental Education*, *73*(9), 1107–1117. www.jdentaled.org/content/73/9/1107.full.pdf+html

Jewell, R. T., McPherson, M. A., & Tieslau, M. A. (2013). Whose fault is it? Assigning blame for grade inflation in higher education. *Applied Economics*, *45*(9), 1185–1200. https://doi.org/10.1080/00036846.2011.621884

Jones-Schenk, J., & Harper, M. G. (2014). Emotional intelligence: An admission criterion alternative to cumulative grade point averages for prelicensure students. *Nurse Education Today*, *34*(3), 413–420. https://doi.org/10.1016/j.nedt.2013.03.018

Latif, D. A. (2004). Using the structured interview for a more reliable assessment of pharmacy student applicants. *American Journal of Pharmaceutical Education*, *68*(1), 1–7. https://doi.org/10.5688/aj680121

Lawshe, C. H. (1975). A quantitative approach to content validity. *Personnel Psychology, 28*(4), 563–575. https://doi.org/10.1111/j.1744-6570.1975.tb01393.x

Levashina, J., Hartwell, C. J., Morgeson, F. P., & Campion, M. A. (2014). The structured employment interview: Narrative and quantitative review of the research literature. *Personnel Psychology, 67*(1), 241–293. https://doi.org/10.1111/peps.12052

Lyon, S. R., Trotter, F., Holt, B., Powell, E., & Roe, A. (2013). Emotional intelligence and its role in recruitment of nursing students. *Nursing Standard, 27*(40), 41–46. https://doi.org/10.7748/ns2013.06.27.40.41.e7529

Mayer, J. D., & Salovey, P. (1993). The intelligence of emotional intelligence. *Intelligence, 17*, 433–442. https://doi.org/10.1016/0160-2896(93)90010-3

McQueen, A. C. (2004). Emotional intelligence in nursing work. *Journal of Advanced Nursing, 47*(1), 101–108. https://doi.org/10.1111/j.1365-2648.2004.03069.x

Pau, A., Jeevaratnam, K., Chen, Y. S., Fall, A. A., Khoo, C., & Nadarajah, V. D. (2013). The multiple mini-interview (MMI) for student selection in health professions training: A systematic review. *Medical Teacher, 35*(12), 1027–1041. https://doi.org/10.3109/0142159X.2013.829912

Petrides, K. V., & Furnham, A. (2001). Trait emotional intelligence: Psychometric investigation with reference to established trait taxonomies. *European Journal of Personality, 15*(6), 425–448. https://doi.org/10.1002/per.416

Portney, L. G., & Watkins, M. P. (2013). *Foundations of clinical research: Applications to practice* (3rd ed.). Pearson, Prentice Hall.

Rankin, B. (2013). Emotional intelligence: Enhancing values-based practice and compassionate care in nursing. *Journal of Advanced Nursing, 69*(12), 2717–2725. https://doi.org/10.1111/jan.12161

Romanelli, F., Cain, J., & Smith, K. M. (2006). Emotional intelligence as a predictor of academic and/or professional success. *American Journal of Pharmaceutical Education*, 70(3). https://doi.org/10.5688/aj700369

Salovey, P., & Mayer, J. D. (1990). Emotional intelligence. *Imagination, Cognition and Personality, 9*, 185–211. https://doi.org/10.2190/DUGG-P24E-52WK-6CDG

Schutte, N. S., Malouff, J. M., & Bhullar, N. (2009). The assessing emotions scale. In Stough, C., Saklofske, D., & Parker, J. (Eds.), *The assessment of emotional intelligence* (pp. 119–135). Springer.

Schutte, N. S., Malouff, J. M., Hall, L. E., Haggerty, D. J., Cooper, J. T., Golden, C. J., & Dornheim, L. (1998). Development and validation of a measure of emotional intelligence. *Personality and Individual Differences, 25*, 167–177. https://doi.org/10.1016/S0191-8869(98)00001-4

U.S. News & World Report. (2015). *Best health care jobs*. https://www.usnews.com/info/blogs/press-room/2015/01/13/us-news-announces-best-jobs-of-2015

Victoroff, K. Z., & Boyatzis, R. E. (2013). What is the relationship between emotional intelligence and dental student clinical performance? *Journal of Dental Education, 77*(4), 416–426. https://doi.org/10.1002/j.0022-0337.2013.77.4.tb05487.x

A table of raw scores was added at the request of one reviewer (Table 15.1).

TABLE 15.1 Distribution of EI Admission Essay Scale Scores

Participant	*EI Admission Essay Scale Score*	*Participant*	*EI Admission Essay Scale Score*
1	14*	28	1**
2	13*	29	1**
3	13*	30	1**
4	12*	31	0**
5	11*	32	0**
6	11*	33	0**
7	10*	34	0**
8	10*	35	0***
9	9*	36	0***
10	7*	37	0***
11	6*	38	0***
12	6*	39	0***
13	3*	40	0***
14	3*	41	0***
15	2*	42	0***
16	2*	43	0***
17	2*	44	0***
18	2*	45	0***
19	2**	46	0***
20	2**	47	0***
21	2**	48	0***
22	1**	49	0***
23	1**	50	0***
24	1**	51	0***
25	1**	52	0***
26	1**	53	0***
27	1**	54	0***

* Indicates scores of applicants (n = 18, 33.33%) who answered the question and wrote about an experience of interpersonal conflict.

** Indicates scores of applicants (n = 16, 29.62%) who misinterpreted the question and wrote about an internal conflict that did not involve the ability to interpret and address others' emotions.

*** Indicates scores of applicants (n = 20, 37.03%) who did not answer the question and wrote about their background, achievements, and career goals.

Checklist for the Revision Process

- ☐ Understand that revision is part of the journal submission process.
- ☐ Depersonalize reviewer feedback by separating emotional reactions from reviewer comments that can strengthen the manuscript. Set aside reviewer feedback for a few days until emotional reactions are no longer experienced.
- ☐ Begin to generate ideas for incorporating requested revisions into the next manuscript draft.
- ☐ If uncertainty exists regarding the meaning of reviewer feedback for a specific item, first consult with coauthors and colleagues. The editor should be contacted directly if a specific reviewer comment cannot be interpreted.
- ☐ Once all reviewer comments are understood, identify those revisions that will be addressed and generate ideas about how revisions will be made.
- ☐ Estimate the time needed for revisions, develop a timeline, and adhere to it so that the manuscript can be resubmitted by the appointed due date.
- ☐ Make sure to adhere to the journal's specified word and page counts during the revision process.
- ☐ When the revised manuscript is complete, generate the document listing responses to reviewer comments. List all reviewer comments followed by complete and clear author responses.
- ☐ In the document listing responses to reviewer comments, justify the decision to omit certain reviewer recommendations with a clear explanation that is free from emotional language.
- ☐ Use neutral, positive language in all correspondence and in the responses to reviewer comments.
- ☐ Thank the editor and reviewers for their help in all correspondence and in the document listing responses to reviewer comments.
- ☐ Thoroughly proof the revised manuscript to identify and correct grammatical and stylistic errors, inconsistencies between citations and references, and inconsistencies between text and tables.
- ☐ Once the manuscript is resubmitted, use the journal's online tracking system to determine the status of a manuscript review. Do not contact the editor until 1 month has expired beyond the allotted review time.

References

Gutman, S. A., & Falk-Kessler, J. P. (2016). Development and psychometric properties of the Emotional Intelligence Admission Essay Scale. *Open Journal of Occupational Therapy*, *4*(3), 1–14. http://dx.doi.org/10.15453/2168-6408.1233

Watkins, L. G. (2020). *Foundations of clinical research: Application to evidence-based practice* (4th ed.). F.A. Davis.

CHAPTER 16

Using Artificial Intelligence in Scholarly Writing

Artificial intelligence (AI) is a set of technologies that enable computer systems to learn, reason, problem-solve, and perform a variety of advanced tasks that mimic human intelligence using vast amounts of available data. AI is programmed to acquire information, use algorithms, and produce an outcome. Advanced AI systems can learn from feedback and improve their performance. AI has become an integral part of daily life and a common tool used by writers.

There are strengths and weaknesses in the use of AI for scholarly writing. The strength of AI is that it can quickly gather information from many resources and synthesize that information to answer questions. AI technologies make it easy to search for resources, allowing authors to synthesize information into coherent, rational, and well-written content.

Conversely, AI sometimes generates inaccurate information, referred to in the technological world as "hallucinations." These hallucinations may include both the content of the writing and the citations and references provided by AI that may be inaccurate or nonexistent. For example, a recent study found that the accuracy of generated references for ChatGPT-3.5 and ChatGPT-4.0 ranged from 47% to 60% and 73% to 87%, respectively (Lechien et al., 2024). The system can gather, synthesize, and repeat information, but it does not have the understanding or experiential learning to know if it is generating accurate information.

In addition to not providing accurate information and citations, AI-generated text is created without critical review. In a podcast interview, Sam Altman, the chief executive officer (CEO) of OpenAI, discussed the difference between intelligence and wisdom, stating that generative AI can create information, but it does not have the critical thinking skills and insight required to provide wisdom (Altman, n.d.). Occupational therapy knowledge is created through a wealth of sources, including research, evidence, clinical experience, critical thinking, and judgment. Authors of scholarly work cannot rely on AI to critically evaluate resources, research methods, and results. AI does not discern various sources of information but rather treats all information as valid. Writers must critically review all sources of information.

DOI: 10.4324/9781003734550-16

The lack of critical review should also be considered for programs that use AI to analyze statistical data, such as programs that integrate ChatGPT with Excel to give instant, quick, and swift results. These programs can analyze data, but they cannot give meaning to the numbers. In addition, the programs reportedly make errors in their analyses (Leonhardt, 2024). Researchers need to understand the statistical analyses, ask for analyses that will answer their research questions, and critically review the findings. In addition, authors need to provide meaningful interpretations of statistical analyses using their clinical and research experience.

AI-Assisted vs. AI-Generated

Despite the limits of AI, it can be a useful tool for scholarly writing and publishing. There are two types of AI content: AI-assisted and AI-generated (Bishop, 2023). AI-assisted content includes text and images that were created by an author who then used computer programs to organize and edit the materials. AI-generated content includes text and images that are "created" by computer programs when given prompts. Authors should keep in mind that AI-generated content is not created by the system but rather synthesized from written materials that it collects and combines from written work to which it has access. In other words, the information "generated" by AI is not actually generated, but more accurately can be described as collected. Therefore, authors must be mindful of providing accurate citations of the work of other authors.

There are several opportunities to use AI-assisted and AI-generated content in scholarly writing. AI-assisted technologies are already used extensively in scholarly writing. Writers commonly use AI-assisted technologies for edit suggestions, spelling corrections, and word generation using programs like Grammarly. AI-assisted technologies may also help with wordsmithing content that has been written by the author. Wordsmithing can make the content clearer and more concise.

Acceptable uses of AI-generated technologies include brainstorming ideas and main points, developing outlines for scholarly papers, summarizing the author's written work, and providing examples of writing in a scholarly genre (Dirette, 2024). Brainstorming can help ensure that authors are not missing any main points. Outlines can help organize and guide the content that will be written by the author. Summaries can be used to help identify the main points for an abstract or conclusion. Examples of writing in a scholarly genre can help authors develop their scholarly voice. AI-generated visual information, such as graphs and tables, can also be useful for illustrating the content discussed by the author. See Table 16.1 for a list of acceptable uses of AI-assisted and AI-generated technologies.

Writing Exercises: AI-Assisted and AI-Generated Exercises

1. Write your introductory paragraph. Enter the paragraph into an AI program such as ChatGPT and prompt it to suggest revisions. Review the feedback and make any edits that improve the paragraph.
2. Write an outline of your manuscript. Enter the outline into an AI program such as ChatGPT and prompt the program to make suggestions for additions,

deletions, or reorganization. Review the feedback and make any revisions that improve the outline.

3. Enter your manuscript into an AI program such as ChatGPT. Prompt it to summarize your manuscript. Use the summary to develop your abstract.

TABLE 16.1 Acceptable Uses of AI Technologies

AI-Assisted	AI-Generated
Editing Suggestions	Brainstorming
Spell Correction	Outline Development
Word Generation	Summaries
Wordsmithing	Writing Examples
	Tables and Graphs

Source: Reprinted from Dirette (2024).

Plagiarism and Copyright Issues

A main concern in scholarly publication using AI is the potential for plagiarism. Plagiarism is representing someone else's writing as one's own without proper acknowledgment, and it is considered to be theft of intellectual property. Generative AI, such as ChatGPT, multiplies the potential for plagiarism, sometimes unbeknownst to the author who is using this technology. Generative AI pulls information from a multitude of sources, usually without quotes or citations of the written materials. And, even when asked for citations, it may hallucinate all or parts of the references. For these reasons, authors should avoid using generative AI to write sentences, paragraphs, or any sections of a manuscript. Authors should carefully review all written work on a topic, critique the content of the work, and synthesize the findings of the work of other authors using proper quotations and citations.

Related to plagiarism are ownership or copyright issues. Copyright is intellectual property generated by authors, including written work, graphs, tables, and other visual displays (www.copyright.gov; retrieved December 29, 2025). These works are protected by copyright laws that forbid the use of the intellectual property of others without proper permission or acknowledgment. This applies to published work but also to authors' works that they upload to AI for assistance. They are exposing their work to copyright infringement, as AI will integrate that work with other published and unpublished work to use when answering questions. The *New York Times* recently filed lawsuits against Perplexity, OpenAI, and Microsoft over their use of copyrighted materials (Metz & Grynbaum, 2025). In addition, several high-profile authors and Getty Images have filed similar lawsuits related to the use of copyrighted materials. These lawsuits not only express concern about violations of copyright laws but also about the accuracy of the content and the citations generated by AI. All authors must be concerned about the legality of using generative AI as a resource to assist with writing content for scholarly publication.

Guidelines for Using AI

The following are general guidelines for using AI in scholarly publications. Each journal, editor, or publishing company may have their own set of guidelines for using AI and requests for disclosure of the use of AI. Authors should review those guidelines before submitting their scholarly work. Authors, peer reviewers, and editors need to adhere to a set of ethical and legal standards that ensure the continued publication of scholarly work that is original and accurate. These guidelines are written to help with that process.

A primary issue related to using generative AI technologies is how to cite them. There is a long-standing tradition of using the work of other authors to build a background and a literature review that demonstrates the relationship of scholarly work to the body of knowledge of the profession (Dirette, 2024). When the work of other authors is used, it is acknowledged with citations or with quotes that are cited. Information created by sources like OpenAI's ChatGPT, however, is not readily retrievable from a citation. Each response generated from technologies like ChatGPT is unique, and a different response may be generated from the same question. This differs from published sources and websites like Wikipedia. The American Psychological Association (APA) is currently working to develop guidelines on how to use and cite generative AI (McAdoo, 2023). Some editors have suggested citing these communications as "personal communications," but there is no person with whom the author has communicated. There are currently three options that are considered to be acceptable.

1. Quotations with Citation: Currently, APA recommends that authors use quotes for text that is written by generative AI with an in-text citation and a reference. The in-text citation should be in parentheses: (OpenAI, 2024) or in the narrative: OpenAI (2024). The reference should be formatted as follows: OpenAI. (2024). ChatGPT (Feb 23 version) [Large language model] (https://chat.openai.com/chat (https://chat.openai.com/chat).
2. Appendices: APA also recommends that the author may include the ChatGPT output as an appendix. The appendix should be cited in the text, and the commands used to generate the text should be discussed.
3. Uniform Resource Locator (URL): Another option for citing a chat from generative AI is for the author to create a URL and use that URL to provide a citation. This will make the chat retrievable for review by editors and readers.

The other major issue that requires guidelines is the acknowledgment or disclosure of the use of generative AI technologies. Authors have a couple of options for this, depending on the journal, publisher, and the type of submission. Some editors may want the use of ChatGPT written in the disclosure section of the submission. Others may want this disclosure included in the text of the paper. For research articles, the use of AI for any part of the research process should be acknowledged in the method section. Authors should review and use the guidelines for the source to which they are submitting their scholarly work.

For occupational therapists and assistants who are reading AI-generated content, the veracity of the information needs to be considered. Because AI provides unfiltered information that lacks critical review, scholars, researchers, and clinicians need to provide their own oversight of the information provided. In clinical practice, there are concerns about accountability related to AI-generated information and who will be held accountable for inaccurate information. If a client is misdiagnosed or provided harmful treatments based on AI suggestions, there are questions related to responsibility and liability, especially as this information is difficult to track. Ultimately, the consumer of AI-generated information is responsible for reviewing, analyzing, and critiquing the information accessed and discerning how it can or cannot be used.

Writing Exercises: AI Copyright and Acknowledgment

1. Write an acknowledgment that describes how AI-assisted and AI-generated technologies were used to compose your manuscript.
2. If there is any written content in your manuscript that was AI-generated, put the written content in quotes and generate a citation acknowledging AI.
3. If any graphics in your manuscript were AI-generated, include an acknowledgment below the graphic and cite the AI-generated source.

Conclusion

AI-assistive technologies can help authors edit and clarify their writing, while AI-generative technologies can help them create content. There are, however, several issues that must be considered when using AI for scholarly writing. The veracity of the content and resources is ultimately the responsibility of the authors, and currently, AI generative technologies are fallible. As content experts, authors with their clinical, scholarly, and research experience should not rely on generative AI to replace their experience, knowledge, and insights when writing scholarly manuscripts. When using AI, authors must follow the guidelines of each specific journal or publisher using proper citations and disclosures. Many publishers are using AI detectors, and these detectors are getting more accurate. Manuscripts may be rejected because they are written by AI. To align with publishers' guidelines, avoid copyright infringement, and maintain the integrity of scholarly writing, authors should limit their use of AI to the suggestions in this chapter, critique any content they acquire from AI, acknowledge any use of AI, and cite AI resources.

References

Altman, S. (n.d.). OpenAI CEO on GPT-4, ChatGPT, and the future of AI (No. 367) [Audio podcast episode]. In Lex Fridman Podcast. https://lexfridman.com/sam-altman/

Bishop, T. (2023, September 11). Amazon distinguishes between ai 'generated' and 'assisted' content in new policy for kindle authors. *GeekWire*. www.geekwire.com/2023/amazon-distinguishesbetween-ai-generated-and-assisted-content-in-new-policyfor-kindle-authors/

Dirette, D. P. (2024). Artificial intelligence: Analysis and guidelines for scholarly writing. *The Open Journal of Occupational Therapy*, 12(2), 1–5. https://doi.org/10.15453/2168-6408.2331

Lechien, J. R., Briganti, G., & Vaira, L. A. (2024). Accuracy of ChatGPT-3.5 and -4 in providing scientific references in otolaryngology-head and neck surgery. *European Archives of Oto-Rhino-Laryngology*, *281*(4), 2159–2165. https://doi.org/10.1007/s00405-023-08441-8

Leonhardt, D. (2024, January 4). First drafts. *The New York Times*. https://messaging-customnewsletters.nytimes.com/dynamic/render?campaign_id=9&emc=edit_nn_20240104&instance_id=111653&nl=themorning&paid_regi=1&productCode=NN&regi_id=85233220&segment_id=154223&te=1&uri=nyt%3A%2F%2Fnewsletter%2F2704fe6f-a24f-5faf-891daa4740d346a7&user_id=a083407e782672cd6e2f2eb6c2c71bce

McAdoo, T. (2023, April 7). How to cite ChatGPT. APA Style. https://apastyle.apa.org/print-this. Downloaded October 20, 2023.

Metz, C. & Grynbaum, M. M. (2025). New York Times sues A.I. start-up Perplexity over use of copyrighted work *The New York Times*. www.nytimes.com/2025/12/05/technology/new-york-times-perplexity-ai-lawsuit.html

CHAPTER 17

Ethical Considerations in Publication

Just as there are ethical issues concerning research misconduct (e.g., mistreatment of participants, failure to gain participant consent and institutional review board approval, and fraudulent data analysis and reporting), ethical issues also pertain to publication misconduct. Publication misconduct is the unethical management of manuscript preparation, submission, and publication. This section addresses issues such as plagiarism, dual submissions, inappropriate authorship, copyright violation, and failure to disclose conflict of interest. Some of these activities are erroneously committed by authors due to lack of knowledge. Understanding common acts of publication misconduct will help you avoid these in the publication process.

Authorship

Authorship is the assignment of ownership to a piece of written scholarship. Authorship should be decided in the early stages of a research project, when roles and activities are defined and assigned. The definition and assignment of roles and activities should be recorded in writing and disseminated to all involved parties. The dissemination process of the written record should request that authors respond to any inconsistencies or inaccuracies by a specified date and that receipt of the document (such as through email) serves as an acknowledgement of agreement unless otherwise specified in writing.

Authorship order should also be decided in the early stages of the project in accordance with the rigor of contributions made to the project by each identified author. First authorship is assigned to the researcher who contributes most to the study design, research implementation, and manuscript writing and preparation. Subsequent authorship is then assigned in accordance with each researcher's contributions. When initial authorship identification and order are decided, it must be acknowledged and understood by all authors that authorship may change if researchers cannot fulfill their specified roles or cannot contribute at the level to which they first committed.

DOI: 10.4324/9781003734550-17

The granting of authorship should be made to researchers who contribute substantially to the conception and design of the study, data collection and analysis activities, and manuscript preparation and submission. Honorary authors (i.e., authors who do not contribute to the study and manuscript preparation but who are listed as authors) and ghost authors (i.e., authors who substantially contribute to study conduction and manuscript writing but are not acknowledged) are examples of inappropriate research practices that prevent full transparency and accountability to the scientific community and public. Honorary authors are often used to increase a study's credibility and impact. Ghost authors are commonly used when manufacturers (such as pharmaceutical or medical equipment companies) carry out a study to demonstrate the effect of their products but falsely list academicians as authors. The practice of ghostwriting in healthcare publications also occurs when seasoned mentors design and/or write significant sections of doctoral student dissertations but are not credited. Both instances of ghost authorship involve falsification of intellectual property and prevent full transparency of and accountability for a research study design and findings.

Research doctoral students who are in the process of turning their original doctoral research into published articles should take responsibility for first authorship but also credit mentors with either authorship or acknowledgment depending on the level of the mentors' contributions. Entry-level health care students who implement a faculty member's research study as part of degree requirements may or may not be considered as authors on a submitted research paper. If students worked on some component of the faculty member's research and helped to collect or analyze data without making any other significant contribution to the study design, implementation, or manuscript preparation, students should be acknowledged for their contribution rather than credited with authorship. If students substantially contributed to multiple components of the design, data collection, analysis, and/or manuscript preparation, student authorship should be considered.

Plagiarism

Piracy is the misappropriation of ideas, data, or work as one's own, instead of obtaining permission from or acknowledging the original authors (Committee on Publication Ethics, 2022). Plagiarism is a form of piracy that specifically involves the misappropriation of written work (including images, tables, and figures) as one's own, rather than obtaining permission from or acknowledging the rightful authors. Plagiarism in journal publication is considered to be an egregious violation of intellectual property rights and truthfulness of ownership. Many acts of plagiarism are unintentional and occur as a result of poor research practices. For example, when reviewing the literature on a specific topic, some authors may copy passages from published articles without making notes indicating that the material has been copied verbatim. They may later use that verbatim material because they forgot that the passage was copied and believed it to be their own words. Today many journals use plagiarism check software programs that can identify plagiarized work in the review process.

Many authors have called for greater leniency of plagiarism definitions with regard to their own work. The publishing world and academia now recognize that authors should be able to use and rework their ideas in multiple publications (Columbia University

Libraries, 2024a). Although verbatim sentences and paragraphs from previously published articles should not be used in subsequent manuscripts, authors are able to use similarly written language and ideas to discuss their work in multiple published articles without being accused of plagiarism and without violating copyright laws. Use of the same data set in multiple publications without disclosure, however, is considered to be a form of research misconduct.

Many authors also serve as reviewers for professional journals. Reviewers must maintain high ethical standards and confidentiality and recuse themselves from manuscript reviews that may present conflicts of interest. Reviewers are commonly asked to review papers whose topics match the reviewer's area of expertise. In such cases, it is unethical for reviewers to use data and information obtained from a manuscript review without crediting the original source. Cases have been disclosed in which reviewers who were exposed to new ideas and data as part of the manuscript review process plagiarized such data and ideas in their own work without crediting the original authors and sabotaged the authors' manuscript, causing rejection. When reviewers act unethically, they are removed from journal review boards, can lose their academic positions, and are often informally blackballed from their profession.

Transparent Reporting of Data, Methods, and Conflict of Interest

Transparency in research reporting is critical to maintain credibility and the trust of the scientific community and public. In past decades, the journal publishing world endorsed a third-person writing style that obscured critical details about researcher roles and study methods that could potentially bias results. Today, journal writing endorses a first-person writing style and requires authors to disclose the roles and activities of all researchers in a study so that readers can evaluate the existence of possible bias. The journal world's adoption of formal reporting standards for clinical studies has also facilitated the transparent reporting of research methods and findings.

Key elements of a research manuscript must be reported transparently. Researchers must clearly report the following:

- Whether institutional review board (or ethics committee) approval was obtained or exempted
- Whether participant consent was obtained for adults; parental or guardian consent and child assent were obtained for minors
- Whether consent was obtained for patients whose data were used in a case report
- Whether any adverse events occurred in the study that impacted results or held implications for the use of the intervention with patients
- Whether the full set of data was used as opposed to data from only those participants who were able to tolerate the testing conditions and/or intervention and completed the study
- Whether missing data exist (the protocol for handling missing data must be reported)
- Whether researchers were anonymized to group assignment and study purpose
- Whether the profession, training, and anonymization procedures of the interveners and data collectors were appropriate for study intent
- Whether interveners were also data collectors

- Whether results were discussed only in the context of literature that supported the researchers' findings while ignoring contrary evidence

Additionally, authors must declare all conflicts of interest. A conflict of interest is a circumstance in which a person derives benefit from a particular situation or event, usually at the expense of others. In journal publication, authors may hold personal interest and derive benefit from the findings of a study. Authors' research may be funded by a source that holds a vested interest in a particular outcome. For example, a researcher's study may be funded by a self-care equipment company that will benefit from studies demonstrating the effectiveness of their products with patients. A researcher may earn monetary derivatives from a newly developed clinical product, such as an edema wrap, and hold a vested interest in studies demonstrating product effectiveness. A researcher may have a family member who owns stock in a motorized mobility equipment company and be involved in patient satisfaction research with such equipment. Authors are required to declare such conflicts of interest and the role of funders in research.

Manuscript reviewers must declare conflicts of interest that may exist before accepting review solicitations. For example, reviewers who engage in similar research as that of the manuscript authors and compete for scarce grant funding with that research team should declare a conflict of interest and recuse themselves from review. Reviewers who believe they can identify the authors of a research manuscript with whom they hold professional disagreements should also recuse themselves from review. In general, if as a reviewer you cannot remove your emotions from the review process and produce a neutrally written review—for personal or professional reasons—you should recuse yourself as a reviewer for that paper. Similarly, many journals allow authors to identify reviewers with conflicting interests and request that such reviewers not be solicited for manuscript review.

Dual Submission, Piecemeal Publication, and Reanalysis of Data

Dual submission (also referred to as simultaneous or multiple submission) is the concurrent submission of the same paper to different journals without disclosing that the paper is being reviewed by more than one journal. When authors submit a paper to a journal, they are commonly asked to confirm that the manuscript is original and has not been submitted elsewhere. Dual submission constitutes an ethical breach of the review process because the same research paper cannot be published by multiple journals without the journals' knowledge and agreement of dual copyright status. If authors have submitted a paper to a specific journal and then wish to submit to another instead, the editor of the first journal must be contacted and the manuscript withdrawn from review.

Piecemeal submission is the unnecessary division of one research study into two or more papers to increase publications. If a research study can be published as one paper and fit journal word count limitations, authors should aim to publish the study in its entirety in one journal article. The only instances that warrant multiple publication of the components of one research study occur when the research components can stand alone, when the authors cannot fit the entire elements of a research study into a single manuscript's page length requirement, and when the material is better organized through the presentation of several papers. An example would be a psychometric measurement study of a specific instrument. If multiple psychometric properties (such as interrater reliability, test-retest reliability, content validity, and convergent validity) have been assessed in one study but cannot be adequately presented in one paper, authors may elect to publish results in two papers. When publishing the results of one study in separate papers, authors should always disclose that results were derived from one study and cite the original paper describing the study.

Reanalysis of data is the use of a published data set to answer different research questions presented in a subsequent manuscript. A paper in which published data are reanalyzed to explore new research questions is legitimate when the data set can truly reveal new and important findings and when the authors disclose that the data set has been previously analyzed and published. When already published data sets are reexamined to yield information about the relationships among variables and do not significantly contribute important knowledge to the profession and society, the research appears disingenuous, and authors appear to be "fishing" for additional publications. In reanalysis of data, authors must always clearly disclose that the data have been derived from an already published data set and cite the original journal article.

Copyright

Copyright is the assignment of legal ownership rights to a given work. While authorship denotes the creators of a work, copyright grants owners the ability to publish and reuse the work. It is common for journals to require manuscript authors to sign a copyright agreement transferring ownership rights to the journal. Although the authors maintain their authorship status, they generally lose control over publication of the article. Many academic organizations have challenged the journal publishing world to modify outdated copyright agreements so that manuscript authors have the right to use their work in future educational and scholarly endeavors, control the future use of their work, and facilitate access of their work by members of the scholarly community (Columbia University Libraries, 2024b; Open Access Initiatives of the Max Planck Society, 2025).

The most common rights that authors should seek in journal copyright agreements regarding the future use of their work include the following:

- The right to reproduce and distribute the work in teaching
- The right to reprint sections of the work in future articles or books
- The right to reuse sections of the work in the creation of related or derivative work (e.g., journal articles, books, and professional presentations)
- The right to be credited as the author of original work that has been released in another form
- The right to post journal articles (in preprint or postprint form) to university digital repositories
- The right to post federally funded journal article research (in preprint or postprint form) to federal digital repositories in accordance with governmental policies

Authors should never transfer copyright of their assessments, clinical guidelines, photographs, illustrations, or unique figures that they will likely wish to use again in publication and education. Instead, authors should maintain copyright of these items and grant the journal permission for one-time printing. The U.S. Copyright Act automatically grants copyright ownership of original work without requiring any action from authors, such as copyright registration; however, copyright registration is recommended for items that are potentially marketable, such as clinical assessments and instruments and continuing education course content (United States Copyright Office, 2009). Authors should make sure that the journal identifies the authors as the copyright owners of a specific item in a note published beneath the item. Maintaining copyright of specific materials eliminates situations in which authors lose control of these items and are forced to pay for and seek permission to use their own work.

Anytime that authors wish to reprint already published materials whose copyright is owned by a journal (such as tables, figures, and assessments), authors must obtain permission from that journal. As mentioned in previous sections of this book, quotations should be avoided in scholarly writing with the following exceptions: a quotation from a historical or legal document, a specific definition accepted by the scientific community whose meaning would change if the exact wording were altered, and specific statements made by participants in qualitative studies. If you quote a passage from a published source that is 50 words or more, many journals require permission from the copyright owner.

Checklist for Transparent and Ethical Publication Preparation and Submission

- ☐ Decide who will receive authorship and in what order early in the project.
- ☐ Record authorship designation and order in written form (all authors should maintain a copy).
- ☐ To receive authorship, all authors should have made substantial contributions to the manuscript.
- ☐ Submit the final manuscript version to a plagiarism check software program to avoid inadvertent violations of copyright.
- ☐ Authors who use their own previously published material in future work should not use verbatim sentences; ideas and similar language can be used.
- ☐ Use a first-person writing style and disclose the roles and activities of all researchers in the study so that readers can evaluate the existence of possible bias.
- ☐ For research studies, indicate whether institutional review board (or ethics committee) approval was obtained or exempted.
- ☐ Indicate whether participant consent was obtained for adults and assent for minors.
- ☐ Indicate whether consent was obtained for patients whose data were used in a case report.
- ☐ Report the occurrence of any adverse events in the study that may have impacted results or hold implications for the use of the assessment or intervention with patients.
- ☐ Indicate whether the full set of data was used as opposed to data from only those participants who were able to tolerate the testing conditions and/or intervention and completed the study.
- ☐ Indicate whether missing data exist and describe the protocol for handling missing data.

- ☐ Indicate whether researchers were anonymized to group assignment and study purpose.
- ☐ Describe the profession, training, and anonymization procedures of the interveners and data collectors (in an intervention effectiveness manuscript).
- ☐ Disclose if interveners were also data collectors (in an intervention effectiveness manuscript).
- ☐ Be clear that results were discussed in the full context of literature rather than only literature supporting the findings.
- ☐ All authors must declare any conflicts of interest and describe the funder's role in the research.
- ☐ Submit the manuscript to one journal at a time; indicate that the manuscript is original and is not being reviewed simultaneously by another journal.
- ☐ If the manuscript is based on a larger study or is a component of another study, disclose this to readers and cite the original study.
- ☐ Indicate if the manuscript is a reanalysis of previously published data and cite the original study.
- ☐ All authors should sign the copyright release form and maintain a copy.
- ☐ Make sure that the copyright agreement allows for basic author rights to reuse one's own work in education and derivative work and to post work to open-access repositories.
- ☐ Do not transfer copyright of assessments, clinical guidelines, and unique images if you intend to use these again in other publications. Instead, grant the journal one-time permission to reprint.
- ☐ Make sure to obtain permission to reprint any materials owned by another source.

References

Columbia University Libraries. (2024a). *Fair use.* https://library.columbia.edu/research-teaching/copyright/fair-use.html

Columbia University Libraries. (2024b). *Copyright information.* http://copyright.columbia.edu/copyright/copyright-ownership/overview/

Committee on Publication Ethics. (2022). *Principles of transparency and best practice in scholarly publishing.* https://publicationethics.org/guidance/guideline/principles-transparency-and-best-practice-scholarly-publishing

Open Access Initiatives of the Max Planck Society. (2025). *Berlin declaration on open access to knowledge in the sciences and humanities.* https://openaccess.mpg.de/Berlin-Declaration

United States Copyright Office. (2009). *Copyright basics.* www.copyright.gov/circs/circ01.pdf

Index

Note: Page numbers in *italics* indicate figures on the corresponding pages.

For Product Safety Concerns and Information please contact our EU representative GPSR@taylorandfrancis.com Taylor & Francis Verlag GmbH, Kaufingerstraße 24, 80331 München, Germany

Batch number: 10739917

Printed by Printforce, the Netherlands